DON'T FORGET FIBRE
IN YOUR DIET

Dr Denis Burkitt worked for nearly twenty years as a surgeon in a teaching hospital in East Africa. During this time he described a form of cancer which now bears his name (Burkitt's Lymphoma).

For this and other work he has received honorary degrees, fellowships and awards from many countries. During the last ten years his studies into world wide disease distribution related to diet have received international recognition. He is a Fellow of the Royal Society in Britain, an Honorary Fellow of Trinity College, Dublin and an Honorary Doctor of Science at Leeds University. He has been awarded the Gold Medal of the British Medical Association; the world's two major cancer research prizes in America in 1982 – the General Motors' Mott Award and the Bristol Myers Award; the Paul Ehrlich-Ludwig Darmstaedter Gold Medal from Germany and the Gardiner Award from Canada.

Dr Burkitt has travelled extensively in all five continents, lecturing and collecting information relevant to his research interests. He has co-edited *Treatment of Burkitt's Lymphoma* (1967), *Burkitt's Lymphoma* (1970), *Refined Carbohydrate Foods and Disease* (1975) and *Western Diseases: Their Emergence and Prevention* (1981). He has also written over 250 scientific publications.

Dr Burkitt values his home life far more than the recognition given his scientific work.

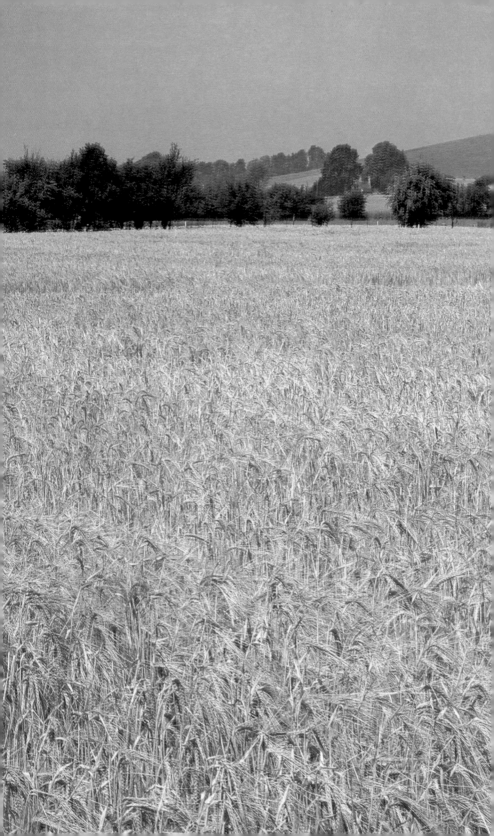

DON'T FORGET FIBRE
IN YOUR DIET
To help avoid many
of our commonest diseases

Fourth, completely revised
and updated edition

Denis Burkitt

CMG, MD, DSc (Hon), FRCS, FRCPI (Hon), FRS

MARTIN DUNITZ

© Dr Denis Burkitt 1979, 1980, 1983
Second edition 1980
Third edition 1980
Revised edition 1981
Reprinted 1982
Fourth, revised edition 1983.

First published in the United Kingdom in 1979
by Martin Dunitz Limited, London.

Cover and studio photographs by Rob Matheson
Text filmset by Bookens, Saffron Walden, Essex

Note. In this book the imperial ounce conversion is used,
that is, 1 oz is taken to be approximately 30 g.

British Library Cataloguing in Publication Data

Burkitt, Denis Parsons
Don't forget fibre in your diet.—4th ed.—
(Positive health guides)
1. High-fiber diet
I. Title   II. Series
613.2'8   RM237.6

ISBN 0-906348-44-7

Printed and bound in Singapore

CONTENTS

To Olive
Without her constant support, the writing of this book would not have been possible.

INTRODUCTION:
THE REASON FOR FIBRE

In recent years doctors and the general public have become increasingly aware of the importance of diet in relation to health. As part of this awareness there has been a great surge of interest in the role of fibre or roughage in our food, and its possible protection against a large number of diseases which are very common in Western countries today.

A striking example of the current recognition of fibre's importance is the Health Education Council of Great Britain's 1982 conclusion that: 'All in all fibre is the single most important form of food likely to be lacking in your everyday diet.' And the same year the following quote appeared in a highly authoritative document produced by the USA's National Research Council: 'It is highly likely that the United States will eventually have the option of adopting a diet that reduces the incidence of cancer by approximately one-third.' The purpose of this book is to suggest that the same would apply to an even greater extent to many common Western diseases other than cancer.

Fibre is the part of food which is not digested by intestinal secretions. Whereas protein, fats and carbohydrates are almost entirely absorbed in the small intestine, fibre passes through to the large intestine almost unchanged. Here much is broken down by bacteria.

Nutrition is derived almost exclusively from the proteins, fats and carbohydrates in the foods we eat. Between them these groups of foods provide nutrients that include vitamins and minerals, materials for growth and repair of body tissue and of course energy. Fibre does none of these things, so although it is present in all plant foods, its significance has been ignored. And yet, if you think about it, there must be a role for a food that does what no other food can do – passing through the upper part of the gut, known as the small intestine, to enter the large intestine more or less in its original state. What, for instance, does its presence do to the contents of the large intestine? This is answered by the fact that it has recently been authoritatively stated that every activity, chemical, physiological, bacteriological and other, that can be measured in the large bowel is affected in a major way by the amount of fibre present in the bowel content. In view of this recognition of the supreme importance of fibre it is sad to reflect that it is the only component of our food that has been deliberately removed (by planned milling policy). This tragic step was the result of ignorance of the nature and properties of fibre that will be discussed in this book.

The question regarding the function of fibre is concerning many scientists today; therefore, in writing this book I have tried to set out in clear language the scientific evidence that has led to the change in attitude with regard to the importance of fibre. I will describe how the implications of this new awareness can be practically applied, with simple, everyday dietary suggestions for protection against some of the most common Western diseases, including constipation, diverticular disease, hiatus hernia, appendicitis, varicose veins, piles, diabetes, obesity, coronary heart disease, bowel cancer and gallstones.

In writing this book, I have deliberately not set out to make it a general work on diet, a task for which I would be unqualified. Instead I have concentrated on this component of food which has been almost totally neglected and have largely confined myself to aspects of nutrition in the study of which I have been personally involved. It is not a good policy to make supposedly authoritative statements without sufficient authority. Regrettably, dogmatic recommendations have often been made by those who are not qualified to do so.

Fortunately my medical background has given me particular opportunities to work in the field of dietary fibre. For twenty years I worked as a surgeon in Africa and during part of this time, and for the sixteen years since leaving Africa, I have been intensively studying on a worldwide basis the geographical distribution of many non-infectious diseases, including all those that will be discussed in this book. Initially my work was limited to cancer but during the last fifteen years I have been collecting material from all over the world on the geographical and cultural distribution of the characteristically Western diseases listed in Chapter 3.

Studies of the geographical distribution of these diseases have made it clear that many of them are rare and some of them virtually unknown among traditionally-living peoples. There is also no evidence that these diseases were other than relatively rare even in Western countries before the present century.

There are, of course, many differences between the life-styles of traditionally living communities and of our own; but there is strong evidence that dietary factors play a predominant role in causing many of these diseases. It is likely that there are multiple causes of each of them and other factors that may be protective against them. Although particular aspects of diet will be emphasized in this book, it is important to remember that it is the whole way of life rather than any single aspect that distinguishes traditional from advanced societies.

Some people have, from time to time, placed undue emphasis on one particular aspect of diet, but the general consensus of informed scientific opinion would agree that the most harmful change that has occurred in Western diets over the past century has been the partial replacement of carbohydrate foods, such as bread and other cereals, by an increased consumption of fat, and of animal fat in particular. Moreover, many carbohydrate foods which were previously eaten with their natural fibre content intact are now consumed largely depleted of their fibre.

One of the first to recognize a relationship between refined carbohydrate foods and disease was Dr T.R. Allinson who, in an essay written nearly a century ago, related not only constipation but also piles (haemorrhoids) and varicose veins to an insufficiency of fibre in the diet. Sir Robert McCarrison, early in the 1900s, warned of the dangers of over-processing food. These observations did not receive serious attention until Surgeon Captain T.L. Cleave, a British naval physician with perceptive genius, persuasive argument and irrefutable logic not only linked together a number of diseases of unknown cause but presented compelling evidence that each of them might be only a different result of a common cause – the consumption of over-refined carbohydrate foods. Captain Cleave demonstrated dramatically the beneficial effect of bran in combating constipation when he was chief medical officer and responsible for the health of the crew of the battleship *King George V* during the Second World War. It was he who first persuaded me of the profound influence of diet on patterns of disease.

In his book *The Saccharine Disease* he described his conviction that many of the characteristically Western diseases might be caused by over-consumption of refined carbohydrate foods, and of sugar in particular, hence the name saccharine meaning 'related to sugar'. This study involved writing letters in longhand to thousands of doctors throughout the world, and thus amassing information on the geographical distribution of various diseases. The data collected compelled the conclusion that the refining of carbohydrate foods might be to a large extent responsible for many diseases characteristic of modern Western culture.

Meeting Captain Cleave was one of the most important occasions in my professional life. Background knowledge of disease patterns in the Third World enabled me to recognize instantly the undeniable truth and logic of his ideas. I also had unique opportunities through medical contacts in much of Africa and Asia to confirm or deny statements he had made, and as will be shown later in this book, the mass of opinion endorsed his conclusions with regard to the relationships between Western diets and Western diseases. Most of the medical profession at that time viewed Captain Cleave's ideas with scepticism, and conse-quently his evidence was rejected without proper consideration.

The recognition given by the medical profession to my earlier work, describing a form of cancer to which my name was given (Burkitt's Lymphoma), provided me with opportunities that would not otherwise have been offered to communicate the concepts of Captain Cleave and others. Moreover, the numerous worldwide contacts I had established for collecting data on cancer distribution provided unique opportunities for testing the validity of these ideas. I was able for example to check the frequency of occurrence of specific diseases in different parts of the world by sending and receiving monthly questionnaires to over 140 rural hospitals in Africa and India.

The original ideas put forward by Cleave and others will stand as landmarks in medical history but details have been, and will continue to be, altered in the light of ever-emerging new facts. Further studies on the influence on health of refining carbohydrate foods have increasingly shifted the blame more on to a reduced fibre intake than to increased sugar consumption, though both are important. Many of the conclusions drawn from evidence currently available and presented in this book are still hypotheses. These may well be changed following further research and future findings. Yet most of those that remain in the state of hypothesis are strengthened by the fact that no alternative theories have yet been put forward that are consistent with the geographical and socio-economic distribution of these diseases or can explain the tendency for more than one of them to occur together in individual patients.

It is not uncommon for people who write on health and other subjects to begin with an emotionally derived conviction and then selectively to look for evidence which will support their preconceived opinions. I have a card on my desk with the all-too-common attitude printed on it, 'My mind is made up, don't confuse me with facts.' Even scientists with commendable enthusiasm can fall into this trap, and I am far from immune, although acutely aware of the difference between provisional hypothesis and proven fact.

In order to emphasize the weight of evidence showing the dominant role of dietary factors as a cause of certain diseases the next two chapters will deal with the principles of the interpretation of this evidence. The techniques of epidemiology, by which is meant the geographical and socio-economic distribution of a disease, and the relationships between a disease and particular factors in the environment will be outlined.

Some readers may prefer to move straight on to the main argument of this book – the relationship between a deficiency of fibre in diet and some of our commonest diseases. If you are less interested in finding out how scientists examine these subjects than in the conclusions they reach, skip the next two chapters and go straight to Chapter 3.

1 WHAT CAUSES DISEASE?

Where we are and what we are

The vast majority of illnesses are the result of where we are, and the environmental circumstances that surround us, rather than of any inherent defect in our make-up. We are constantly being influenced by a multitude of seen and unseen things – the sun's rays, the food and drink that enter our body and the air we breathe. In addition we are exposed to hostile attack by other creatures and also by our fellow men.

On the other hand we have, built into our systems, elaborate and beautifully designed mechanisms to counter the attack of a huge variety of bacteria and parasites that may invade our bodies. We are partially protected by the pigment in our skin from the effects of excessive sun radiation and by the reflex mechanisms that take instantaneous and automatic action at the approach of danger. An example is the way we immediately close our eyelids when anything touches our eyes.

People of different ethnic groups usually suffer from the same diseases when living in the same environment, whereas those from the same groups, if living in different environments, suffer from different diseases, depending on the harmful factors to which they are exposed in these environments. However, different ethnic groups and different individuals are more or less susceptible to particular injurious elements in their environment. The Chinese people, for example, no matter where in the world they live, are more likely to develop a form of cancer that grows at the back of the throat and there is some statistical evidence that Indians are more likely to suffer from coronary heart disease than are Western populations when exposed to the same risk factors. An

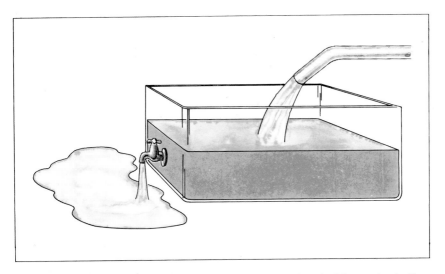

The risk of developing disease, represented by the level of the water in the tank depends on the relative amounts entering and leaving, depicting causative and protective factors.

example of protection conferred by genetic factors is the reduced risk of developing malaria observed in some Africans due to an abnormality of the red blood cells.

The balance of health

Too often disease is viewed merely as the result of harmful influences, while factors that protect from disease are overlooked. Both sickness and health are dependent on a balance between beneficial and harmful influences, between the effectiveness of the things that attack us and the ability of our bodies to defend themselves. The situation can be compared to a conflict between two opposing armies. If one of the armies is depleted, it will have an effect on the outcome of the battle, as will augmenting the opposing forces. Although many of our general protective mechanisms against disease are inbuilt before birth, we can develop particular defences against specific diseases as a result of successfully combating attacks by the organisms which produce these diseases.

The balance between attacking and defending forces in our bodies can be compared to a water tank with one pipe supplying water to it and another draining water from it (above). The level of the water in the tank

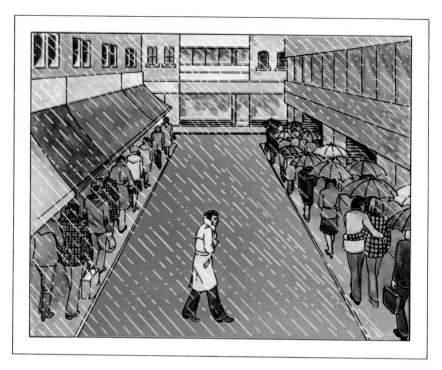

depends on the relative amount flowing from each tap. The water entering can be taken to represent the cause of a disease, the outflow the protective mechanisms, and the level of water the risk of developing disease. The higher the level – the greater the risk. Increasing the inflow or reducing the outflow will have the same effect and vice versa.

Bodies like the Food and Drugs Administration in the United States are right to be careful to ensure that potentially harmful substances are not added to food, but how much thought is given to the removal of potentially protective components of food?

All animals, including man, tend to adapt to any hostile elements in the environment in which they live, so that in time they develop mechanisms which protect them against these dangers. For example, animals develop body colours which blend with their environment and thus provide protection through camouflage. In a similar way polar animals develop furry coats that insulate them against the cold.

Men or animals who are not normally exposed to certain hostile environments do not require protection against them. They are like the men on the left of the illustration (above) who are under shelter, so do not require umbrellas to protect them from the rain. Rain is falling around those on the right of the illustration but these people remain dry, that is, disease free, because they have acquired protection in the form of umbrellas. If a man without an umbrella walks from shelter into the rain he gets wet. The rain in the illustration represents an environment capable of causing a disease to develop. The people under shelter are not exposed to the environment so remain dry, that is, disease free. Those who are in the harmful environment of the rain and have acquired the protective immunity of the umbrellas also remain dry, that is, free of disease. Those who go into the harmful environment without this protection get wet, that is, they will develop the disease.

As mentioned earlier, some people, because of their genetically inherited make-up, are more susceptible to certain disease-producing influences than are others. If once again we compare the environment in which we find ourselves to rain, and our protection against disease to umbrellas, our chances of keeping dry will depend not only on the possession of an umbrella but also on its size, that is, the extent of the protection that we have against the hostile environment. An understanding of this principle of adaptation to environment is very relevant to the main argument of this book which deals with the diseases characteristic of modern Western man.

We have already seen that most disease is caused by environment, and even defects present at birth can be the result of some harmful factor during the baby's development in the womb. A good example of this is the tragedy of the deformities caused to the unborn child by the mother taking the drug thalidomide. There are also a few diseases which are transmitted genetically from parent to child.

Changing patterns of disease

Environmental causes of disease are very varied. The major cause is infection from bacteria and parasites of different kinds. Causes of the different infective diseases are now largely known, and consequently energetic measures have been highly successful in controlling most of them. As a result in Western countries the pattern of disease has dramatically changed over the past century. A hundred years ago by far the commonest causes of illness and death were infective diseases such as pneumonia, gastro-enteritis, diphtheria, tuberculosis and meningitis.

Deaths from these causes are relatively rare today. These and other infective diseases are, however, still the major cause of sickness and death in the Third World.

The major health hazards, providing the commonest causes of death in Western countries today, are the non-infective diseases whose causes are still usually unknown. These include certain types of cancer, arterial disease and other so-called 'degenerative' diseases. They are, however, all rare in Third World countries, even among the elderly. Because of this new knowledge the name 'degenerative' hardly seems appropriate.

Weighing up the causes

It is important to recognize that many different factors may contribute to the cause of any one disease. Coronary heart disease is probably a good example. Male sex, high blood pressure, smoking and consumption of large quantities of fat and cholesterol are regarded as high-risk factors, whereas exercise and fibre-rich cereal foods have been claimed to be protective. It is possible to reduce the risk of a disease by getting rid of a major cause. For example, giving up smoking will drastically reduce the occurrence of lung cancer but not totally eliminate it as there are other causes. All the effects of a common cause are associated with each other. Consequently, associations found between diseases suggest they share a common cause (see diagram opposite).

The situation can also be compared to the balance of weighing scales. On one side you have the causative factors of disease, represented by one pan of the scales. On the other, there are the various protective factors. When the causative ones outweigh the protective factors, forcing the first pan down, disease occurs.

Not only can several different factors contribute to the cause of a single disease, but a single factor may contribute to the cause of a number of apparently different diseases, which in certain circumstances may be viewed as different aspects of a single disease – as they share a common cause. For example, typhoid fever, which used to be common in Western countries and is still common in tropical regions, can show itself in many different forms, some appearing long after the acute phase of the disease is over. It gives rise not only to fever, a skin rash, abdominal pain and changes in the blood in its early stages, but subsequent effects include changes within the bones, gall-bladder

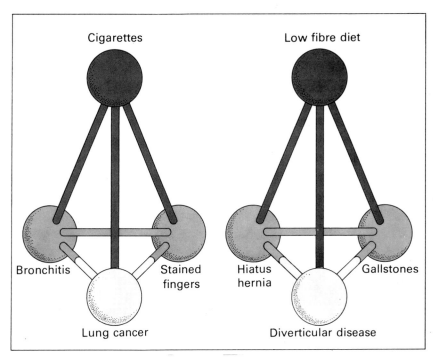

The effects of a common cause are associated.

disease and arthritis. Each of these might well have been considered to be a different disease before the underlying cause of each – the bacteria responsible for causing typhoid fever – was identified. Once the basic cause had been identified, it became possible to protect against it. Not only can one factor be a cause of a number of different diseases but the same can apply to factors protecting us against several diseases.

Later in this book I will show how relevant these basic principles and simple illustrations are to discovering the causes of, and the means of prevention from, some of our commonest diseases. It has been found more acceptable to consider fibre a protection against many diseases than to view lack of fibre as a cause of them, although both concepts are equally valid.

2 HOW ENVIRONMENT PLAYS A PART

Life expectancy at birth in Western countries is much greater today than it was a century or more ago. This is much more the result of clean water supplies, satisfactory sewage disposal, adequate nutrition, ample clothing and shelter than of therapeutic medicine. Although infant mortality has fallen enormously during this century (see diagram opposite), life expectancy in middle age has scarcely increased. This is largely because relatively new diseases have taken the place of infective diseases as a major cause of death.

In 1950 less than one medical prescription was issued per person per year in Australia; by 1975 the figure had risen to over ten. Yet during this time there has been no appreciable change in life expectancy after middle age in spite of the enormously increased availability of potent drugs to combat infection.

It is true that new drugs such as certain antibiotics played a significant role in treating tuberculosis – once a major scourge in Western countries, but it is important to appreciate the manner in which infective disease, such a major cause of death in the past, was conquered in Western countries. The factors most responsible were increased resistance to disease as a result of improved nutrition, and reduced contact with disease-causing organisms effected by the supply of clean water and milk and adequate sewage disposal. Immunization contributed in the case of some diseases like diphtheria, poliomyelitis and whooping cough.

The important lesson learned is that reductions in mortality rates were not significantly influenced by treatment because the major

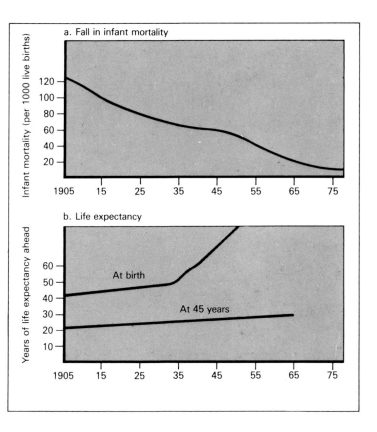

a	The fall in infant mortality from 1905 to 1975.

b	The higher life expectancy at birth due to the fall in infant mortality from 1905 to 1975, but showing the minimal increase in life expectancy at 45 years old.

reductions had occurred before any effective treatment became available. With the exception of diseases conquered by immunization, reduction of disease has almost always followed identification and reduction or removal of causative factors.

In Western countries today diseases produced by bacterial infections are no longer the major cause of death as they were a century and more ago. Their place as major causes of death and disability has been taken by the so-called 'degenerative' diseases. Fortunately, as will be shown in this chapter, a very useful method of looking at modern disease has been evolved which points the way to a better understanding of the underlying causes of non-infective diseases.

Geographical distribution – a clue to the cause of disease

Most diseases are caused by harmful factors in the environment, so it follows that the high incidence of a disease in a certain area or among a particular group of people may point to some local causative factor. Low prevalence rates may reflect minimum activity of causative factors or alternatively the presence of protective factors. If people of different races in a particular environment get a certain disease, but in a different environment are all free from this disease, it can be concluded that the principal cause of the disease lies in the environment and not in the genetic make-up of the different people.

The study of the geographical or socio-economic distribution of disease is called epidemiology. One of the most fruitful ways of discovering the cause of a disease is by studying its pattern of distribution and then considering possible disease-causing factors with the same distribution. One classic example of this approach is John Snow's discovery of the cause of cholera. In a cholera epidemic Snow plotted on a street map of London the distribution of cholera cases and then searched for some factor that was common to them all and which might link them together. He found that they all drew their water from the same pump in Broad Street. The water from this pump was drawn from the River Thames below the entry of sewage disposal and was thus contaminated with human excreta. Not till many years later was the organism responsible for cholera identified.

Another example is Sir Percival Pott's discovery, over a century ago, that many of the elderly men consulting him with skin cancer had been employed as chimney sweeps as young boys. He related the cancer to skin contact with soot-impregnated clothes long before it became known that soot contains substances that can be carcinogens (cancer-forming substances).

It is important to remember that both Snow and Pott recognized causative associations between diseases and particular factors in the environment long before the ways in which they produced disease became understood. They were able to advise means of prevention without waiting until science provided proof that the suspected factors were in fact causes of the associated diseases.

Relationships between diseases

Different diseases may share the same causes and they will consequently tend to occur not only in the same geographical locations, but also in the same individuals. The typhoid fever example, mentioned in Chapter 1, illustrates this. The many different clinical manifestations of the disease associated in the same patients suggested they might share a common cause.

When one disease follows another it is sometimes wrongly assumed that the second is caused by, and is a complication, of the first. An alternative explanation may well be that both diseases are due to a common cause, and that the second to appear requires more time to develop than does the first. It may be that factor X causes disease A, then disease A causes disease B.

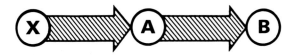

Alternatively, both A and B may be independent results of the common cause of X with A appearing before B.

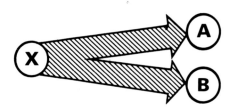

It is also possible that the different causes of two different diseases or groups of diseases may be related to one another, as a result of which the diseases are related because they share a related but not a common cause. Naturally, if you are trying to find factor X you have to look for reasonable links between the environment and diseases represented by A and B. In some countries the increase in lung cancer might be related to the number of television sets, but this does not necessarily imply that television viewing causes lung cancer. To return to our analogy of the pipe filling the tank. A tank may have a pipe leading into it from which no water is flowing; therefore this pipe could not influence the water level of the tank. Or the tank can have a pipe leading into it from which water is flowing which will influence the water level. The former is a non-causative and the latter a causative relationship.

Age is a factor that determines susceptibility to disease. This is partly because the longer you live the more exposed you are to detrimental factors in the environment and partly because defence mechanisms against disease become weaker in old age. Advancing age makes such an enormous difference in cancer risk that for most forms of cancer the differences observed between young and old people in the same area are much greater than the different incidences for that tumour between the regions where it is least or most prevalent.

It is often incorrectly assumed that because life expectancy at birth in poorer countries may be only forty years this implies that there are few old people. It is, however, mainly the high infant mortality that lowers the average life expectancy at birth rather than death in middle life. Although there are significantly fewer old people in Third World countries than in Western communities there are plenty of them, and the rarity of many of the diseases discussed in this book cannot therefore be explained by a lack of elderly people in the population.

The distribution in the population of people of different ages in India and the United States shows that the lower life expectancy at birth is influenced much more by the high infant mortality than by the premature death of people who survive to adult life. Although there are more old people in Western countries, the proportion of people over fifty is only about two and a half times greater in the United States despite the far greater proportion surviving childhood. If a disease characteristic of old age is, say, three times as common in Western countries as in Third World communities, the age discrepancy might account for it, but certainly not when the discrepancy is between ten and over one hundred times, as it is in the case of many of the diseases discussed in this book. With this in mind, we will, in the next chapter, look at the distribution of some of the typically Western diseases round the world, comparing their occurrence in more developed and in less developed countries.

22

3 CAN SOME OF OUR COMMONEST AILMENTS BE PREVENTED?

Worldwide comparisons

Once you begin to compare the occurrence of some of our most common diseases with their incidence in other parts of the world you start to find dramatic differences. These differences will be described here but possible reasons for these wide variations will be considered in Chapters 4 and 5.

Coronary heart disease

This is the commonest cause of death in Western countries, killing about one man in four. It is also an increasingly important cause of death among older women. It was a rarely reported disease even in Western countries until after the First World War. Coronary heart disease is almost unknown among rural Africans and is uncommon in most rural communities in Asia. In African cities only occasional cases are found and these are always among the most Westernized sections of the community. It was much less common among black than white Americans forty and more years ago, yet black and white Americans living in similar circumstances are comparably affected by this disease today.

Gallstones

Removal of the gall-bladder is currently one of the most frequently performed abdominal operations in Western countries and gallstones have become much commoner during this century. They are exceedingly rare in Africa, where many rural hospitals may not see even one patient with gallstones in ten years.

The Pima Indians in the south-west of the United States have been found to have a higher frequency of gallstones than any other group. Over 70 per cent of Pima Indian women between twenty-five and forty have gallstones. They are present in over 20 per cent of women over the age of thirty in most Western countries. Fortunately most never know they have them, and never get ill.

Diverticular disease of the colon

This is the commonest disease of the large intestine. It is present, though usually without symptoms, in one in ten people over the age of forty, and in one in three over the age of sixty. Even in Western countries it was rarely reported before the late 1920s. Of all the modern diseases this is the rarest in Third World communities. It has until recently been almost unknown in Africa and in Asia. The few cases observed in Asian and African countries have for the most part been in the top socio-economic levels of the community. Only occasional cases are observed even in large university clinics in India.

Appendicitis

This is the most frequent cause for emergency abdominal surgery. About one person in eight has had his or her appendix removed by middle age. As with the diseases listed above, the frequency of appendicitis greatly increased in Western countries during the early years of the present century, before probably reaching a fairly stationary level. It became less common in many European countries during both World Wars when there was strict food rationing. It was almost unknown to doctors in many of the prisoner-of-war camps.

In Africa and Asia appendicitis is a disease of urban populations and of upper socio-economic groups rather than of peasant rural communities. We taught our Ugandan doctors that they should be wary about diagnosing appendicitis in an African unless he could speak English. This was an index of his contact with Western culture!

In the past, when food in British prisons was coarser than that eaten outside, appendicitis was less common among prisoners than in the rest of the population.

Presumably it was not found among American slaves when they were brought from rural Africa, but it had become fairly common among black Americans forty or fifty years ago. Appendicitis is as common now among black as white Americans.

Hiatus hernia

This is an upward protrusion of the top of the stomach into the thoracic cavity through the hole in the diaphragm through which the oesophagus or gullet passes (see page 56). It can be demonstrated in about one in five adults by taking an X-ray after the person has eaten a meal containing barium which is radio-opaque. The majority of patients with hiatus hernia have no symptoms. A number, however, suffer from heartburn owing to the entry of gastric acid into the gullet. This disease is very rare among traditionally living people. A radiological study in West Africa revealed only four cases in over a thousand adults who were carefully examined for the presence of this defect. Similar figures have been reported from other parts of Africa. It is a little commoner in Asian communities but still rare compared with Western countries.

Varicose veins

A community-wide study in Michigan in the United States showed that 44 per cent of women between the ages of thirty and fifty had varicose veins compared to 24 per cent of men in the same group. The same study found 64 per cent of women over fifty had them compared to 42 per cent of men. Varicose veins are much less common in developing countries and are particularly rare among people who have had minimal contact with Western culture. Varicose veins have been estimated to be present in under 5 per cent of rural Africans and Indians. Their prevalence in different groups of Pacific Islands is directly related to contact with Western culture. Varicose veins are even more common among New Zealand Maori women than white women, and equally common among black and white Americans today.

In Asia varicose veins are more common among trishaw riders who ride a tricycle which carries passengers seated behind than they are among barbers who stand at their work. The former are subject to considerable abdominal straining as they pedal. These examples show that environmental factors are more important than genetic ones in causing this disorder.

Piles (haemorrhoids)

These are now viewed in an entirely new and different way from the traditional approach. They are normal structures and it is only the complications that commonly occur, such as bleeding, prolapse and clotting of contained blood that can be considered diseases. These are very common in Western societies but relatively rare in Third World countries.

Large bowel cancer

This is the most common cause of cancer death, second only to lung cancer due to cigarette smoking, in North America and in Britain. There is no other type of cancer so closely related to economic development and our way of life. It is far more common in Western communities than it is in the populations of the Third World.

In North America there are two religious groups who suffer about a third less bowel cancer than other Americans. These are the seventh Day Adventists who are predominantly vegetarian, and Mormons who are not. These two groups also have a much lower risk of developing coronary heart disease and, being non-smokers, are almost completely free from lung cancer.

Although they live in a comparable culture, rural Finns have only about a quarter the incidence of bowel cancer of Copenhagen Danes or New Yorkers.

Breast cancer

This is the commonest cancer affecting women in Western communities, in which it is more often observed in meat-eating people than in vegetarians. It is much less frequent in developing countries.

Diabetes

This can be the most common disorder of the endocrine glands. It is present, though not necessarily detected, in about 5 per cent of the American population and about 15 per cent over sixty. The percentage in Britain appears to be slightly lower. It has not yet been reported among any pure-blooded hunter-food gatherers, such as African bushmen, or in Eskimos (living in their traditional manner). One of the most striking examples of the way in which this disease is related to a modern Western life-style is provided by the little island of Nauru in the Pacific.

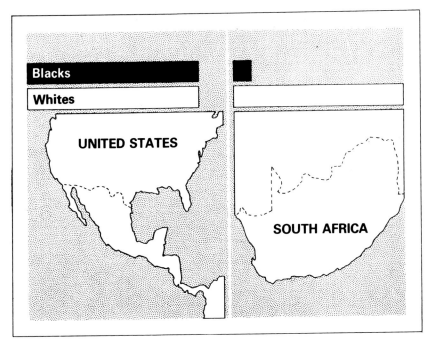

The blocks represent the occurrence of the diseases described in this chapter. They occur as frequently among black Americans as among white Americans and white South Africans. Black South Africans are rarely affected.

A few years ago it was discovered that the whole island was covered with phosphates, obviously of great economic value. As a result its people are now among the wealthiest in the world after the Arabs in the Middle East. They import Western-type food, lead a leisurely life, and already over 40 per cent of the population over the age of twenty suffers from diabetes, whereas once the incidence of the disease was as low as it is in other Pacific islands. They are increasingly suffering from appendicitis, another disease to emerge relatively early after impact with Western culture. Coronary heart disease and gallstones will almost certainly emerge in time. Diseases like hiatus hernia and diverticular disease will not be expected until after at least a generation.

Another striking example of the effect of environment on diabetes is provided by the Indians in South Africa whose forebears emigrated from south India. They now get about ten times as much diabetes as Indians who live in India.

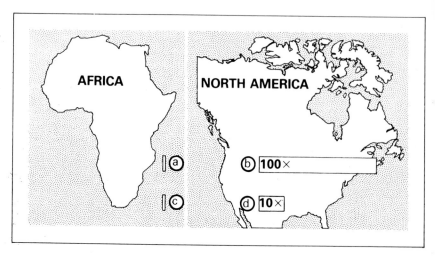

Blocks a and b represent the occurrence of coronary heart disease, diverticular disease, gallstones, appendicitis and hiatus hernia in areas like North America b and rural Africa a. They occur about 100 times more frequently in b than a. Varicose veins, piles, large bowel cancer, diabetes and obesity, represented by blocks c and d occur about ten times more frequently in areas like North America than rural Africa.

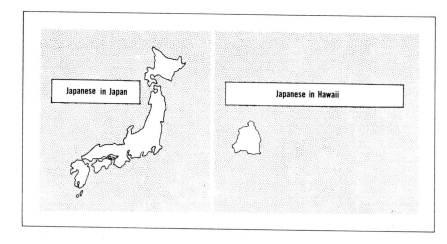

These diseases were relatively rare in Japan until after the Second World War. They are still much less common there than in the US, but are increasing in Japanese cities.

Within a generation of Japanese emigrating to Hawaii the occurrence of these diseases had become comparable to that among other Americans.

Obesity

At least 40 per cent of middle-aged adults in North America and Western Europe are overweight. This is rarely a problem in tribal communities among whom weight increases little after early adult life. Indeed in such communities average body weight actually falls during middle age whereas it rises in all Western communities.

All the diseases listed in this chapter have been until recently rare among black South Africans but affect white South Africans to approximately the same extent as Americans. Diabetes and obesity are now common in the black community. Yet in the United States they affect blacks and whites to a comparable extent. They were presumably as rare or rarer among American slaves as they are today in the parts of Africa from which the slaves came. Forty or more years ago the diseases for which information is available were much less common among black than white Americans, but both groups are equally affected today.

These diseases were uncommon in Japan until after the Second World War, but are now increasing rapidly. Japanese who emigrated to Hawaii and California and adopted an American way of life have, within a generation, become almost equally prone to develop these diseases as other Americans (left, below).

From the above information we are forced to draw the inescapable conclusion that these common diseases are primarily the result of a man-made environment rather than genetic in origin. If we could only identify and eradicate or minimize their causes these diseases would be largely preventable.

Not only do they have similar geographical and socio-economic distributions, but many of them tend to occur together in individual patients. These observations suggest that the diseases described all share some common or related causes although these need not be their only causes. Alternatively some factor in the environment may provide protection against each of these diseases.

In the following chapters we will consider which factors in these contrasting environments are most likely to be responsible for causing or protecting against these diseases. The first step in the prevention of any disease is, of course, identification of its cause, and a study of these possible factors will give us some clues as to means of prevention.

4 LOOK TO YOUR DIET

Changing eating patterns

In the last chapter it was shown that a formidable list of diseases is common in Western countries but rarely found in less developed parts of the world. Even in Western countries many of them have only become widespread during the last sixty or so years. Therefore the main causes must lie in some aspects of our modern way of life.

I will show in later chapters that many of the diseases mentioned are related either directly or indirectly to the behaviour of the gut (known as the intestinal tract) and the nature of the intestinal content. In view of the staggering disparity in the frequency of these diseases in Western and Third World countries, it seems logical as a next step to compare the usual dietary habits in the places where they are rarely found with those of communities most affected.

When food is prepared in a simple way such as grinding grain by hand between two stones, or pounding it in a wooden tub, and large amounts of the product are then eaten with little extracted or removed from it, all the diseases mentioned are relatively rare. The earliest changes in diet that take place in Third World countries as they begin to develop economically are usually the introduction of sugar, sweetened drinks and white bread or white rice in place of the minimally processed carbohydrate foods that previously provided the staple diet. The eating pattern changes towards the style of a typical Western diet where fat plays a prominent role, sugar intake increases (pages 31 and 34) and consumption of little-processed starchy foods such as whole grains and potatoes is considerably reduced.

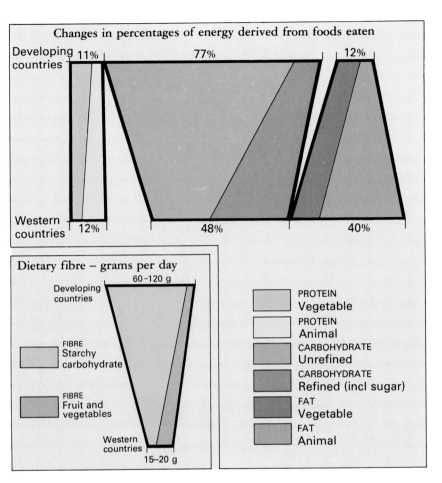

Changes in percentages of energy derived from foods eaten

Developing countries: 11% | 77% | 12%

Western countries: 12% | 48% | 40%

Dietary fibre – grams per day

Developing countries: 60–120 g
Western countries: 15–20 g

FIBRE Starchy carbohydrate

FIBRE Fruit and vegetables

PROTEIN Vegetable

PROTEIN Animal

CARBOHYDRATE Unrefined

CARBOHYDRATE Refined (incl sugar)

FAT Vegetable

FAT Animal

Above: The relative proportion of energy (calories) provided by protein, carbohydrate and fat in Third World compared to Western countries.
*Below:*Changes in fibre intake both overall and in source.

This means there are fundamental changes in the proportions of energy derived from the three main food components: protein, carbohydrate and fat (see above). The differences between the food consumed in Western communities today and that eaten by rural populations in the Third World are similar to the differences between Western diets today compared to the food our ancestors ate a century or more ago.

The proportion of energy derived from protein is fairly constant, usually varying somewhere between 10 and 15 per cent. Its nature, however, changes from being mainly derived from vegetable foods in developing countries to being largely of animal origin in more affluent societies. Fat intake rises with economic development so that Western communities eat three or four times as much fat as do people in poorer countries. In addition its nature changes, as in the case of protein, with animal fat largely replacing vegetable fat.

Along with the rise in fat consumption goes a change both in overall carbohydrate intake and also in the kind of carbohydrates eaten. In rural communities in the Third World carbohydrate provides between 70 and 80 per cent of energy, and is consumed with its full complement of fibre, the indigestible portion consisting largely of plant cell walls. In Western countries the fibre content has been largely extracted in the manufacture of sugar and highly refined white flour. The latter has replaced brown and wholemeal flour which are rich in fibre. Modern milling methods strip away the outer layers of the grain. Refined sugar, which is almost entirely composed of calories, and white flour now provide much of our reduced carbohydrate consumption. The average annual sugar intake in Western countries of about 100 lb (45 kg) is about ten times that in poorer countries. Consumption of potatoes has also fallen in Western countries.

The significance of fibre

The food component that changes most with adoption of Western dietary habits is the indigestible fibre. Four or five times as much fibre is consumed by rural communities in the Third World as by Western populations, the former consuming some 2–4 oz (60–120 g) and the latter only around ½ oz (15–20g) per person daily. In Western countries fibre is derived mainly from fruit and leaf vegetables whereas in Third World countries it is mostly provided by cereal foods, root vegetables and legumes.

As in the case of fibre the nature of protein consumed also differs between poorer and richer communities. Whereas total protein intake in affluent communities is only moderately more than in poor countries, the proportion derived from animal sources is seven times greater. While fat intake in the Western diet is about three times greater than that of poor countries, the proportion derived from animal sources is eight times greater. The difference in sugar intake can be as great as tenfold.

It will be seen that the intake of fibre and starch has been reduced as that of fat and sugar has increased (see page 91). As consumption of fats and oils has increased the consumption of grains and potatoes has decreased (see page 34).

The fibre reduction is relatively greater than the carbohydrate reduction. When carbohydrate foods provide a high proportion of the total calories consumed in the daily diet they are lightly processed foods which are relatively rich in fibre. When they provide a smaller proportion of energy more of them are highly processed cereal foods, such as white flour or white rice, with less fibre, and sugar which is entirely depleted of its fibre.

As pointed out in the last chapter, fibre from fruits and vegetables has, over the past century, increased in Western countries whereas fibre from cereals has decreased (see page 35). Although the total consumption of fibre has not altered greatly in Western countries, recent research has indicated that cereal fibre present in brown or wholemeal bread, coarse oatmeal, rye crispbread, breakfast cereals, brown rice and bran is more likely to be effective in preventing certain diseases than an equal amount of fibre derived from fruit and vegetables. This will be discussed in more detail in Chapter 12.

As an example of the effect of this difference, studies of the diet of South African Bantu have shown that their fibre intake is over four times that of Western communities. This would almost certainly be true of all African communities in sub-Saharan Africa, among whom virtually all the Western diseases are invariably rare.

We have already seen that fat and carbohydrate intake are reciprocally related and this is an exceedingly important fact. Together they provide between 85 and 90 per cent of energy in most communities, so that a high fat diet is inevitably a low carbohydrate diet and vice versa (see page 35). Since reduction in carbohydrate is accompanied by a much greater reduction in fibre, fibre intake and fat intake are almost always inversely related. As intake of fat goes up, that of carbohydrate and fibre goes down.

In Western countries today sugar, which is pure energy, accounts for 40 per cent of our energy derived from carbohydrate foods. Foods composed mainly of white flour, sugar and fat have to a large extent replaced the fibre-rich cereals; tubers, including potatoes and parsnips; and legumes, including peas and beans. All these could be easily stored

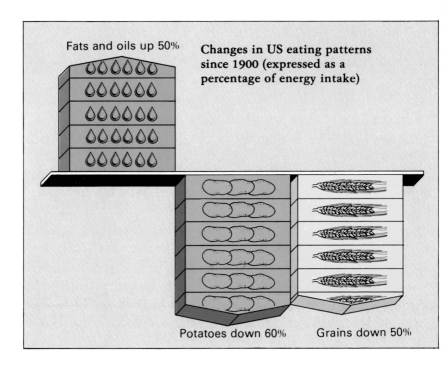

Fats and oils up 50%

Changes in US eating patterns since 1900 (expressed as a percentage of energy intake)

Potatoes down 60%   Grains down 50%

and were eaten in larger quantities previously. Now approximately half of our reduced fibre intake comes from fruit and vegetables.

Because of the reciprocal relationship between fat and fibre intake, epidemiological evidence that points to an increase in fat consumption as a cause of any disease must point equally strongly to a decrease in fibre. Neither of these opposite sides of the coin should be viewed in isolation. The more bulky fibre-rich foods you eat the less fat you will be consuming, and vice versa. At its simplest, if you eat more fibre-rich foods they are bulkier and fill the stomach up while providing less energy than foods that are rich in calories like sugar and fat. How this happens will be shown in Chapter 11 when we come to look at some of the factors responsible for obesity.

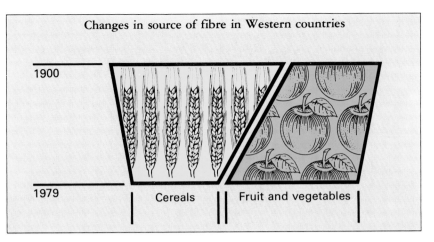

The proportion of fibre provided by cereals has been reduced, while that from fruit and vegetables has increased.

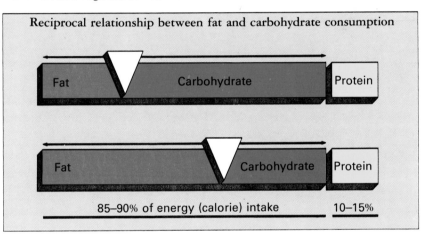

5 FIBRE – THE FORGOTTEN FACTOR

We have now looked at the main energy-providing components of our diet – protein, fat and carbohydrate. There are of course other nutritional requirements such as vitamins and small quantities of minerals such as zinc, iron and calcium.

Nutritionists have given much thought to these three major energy-containing, calorie-rich components of food. The less nutritious portion, the fibre, has been misunderstood, neglected and rejected for too long. Because it was previously thought to provide no energy, fibre had been viewed as being of no value in food and its removal was believed to improve the quality of plant foods and of cereals in particular. It was in fact regarded as a contaminant and consequently discarded to be used as animal feed. Although some individuals have in the past recognized this approach as being wrong, only in recent years has the fallacy of this assumption been scientifically demonstrated and consequently widely recognized among food scientists.

What is fibre and why is it important?

Fibre is the skeleton of the plant, without which no flower or tree would be able to stand upright. The walls of every cell are composed of fibre. The contents of a cell are the nutrients, the cell wall is their carton or container. Nutritionists have examined in detail the content but ignored the carton (page 37).

The fibre is more abundant on the outside of seeds, fruits, legumes (peas and beans) and other foods than on the inside, and with the

Plant cell

Grain of wheat

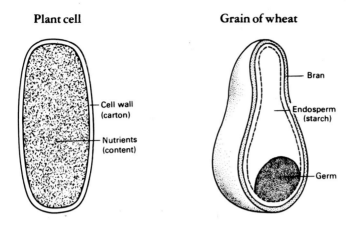

removal of the outside layers in milling and peeling much of the all-important fibre is discarded. Fibre is also removed when the content of cells is extracted and the cell wall removed, as in the extraction of sugar from cane or beet; also when vegetable oils and fats are extracted from oil seeds, cereals and nuts.

Fibre is not a single substance, but is basically a mixture of three main groups of substances. One is cellulose (a polysaccharide), another is lignin, which provides the woody part of plants. It is the only part of fibre that is not carbohydrate. There is a separate group of poly-saccharides composed mainly of sugars, called pentoses, but including pectin (the setting agent in jams) and also gums, which are present in certain beans. The entire mix has been likened to ferro-concrete used for building construction, with cellulose representing the long straight iron bars; pentoses the branched-rods; the more soluble pectins and gums corresponding to the cement; and the lignin forming the tough outer covering.

It is interesting to note that at one time fibre was almost entirely equated with cellulose whereas it is now recognized that this is one of its less important constituents. The use of the term 'crude fibre' denoted only that part of plant food which was not broken down by boiling successively in weak acid and weak alkali. This, in fact, measured only part of the cellulose and part of the lignin (which gives wood its hardness), and none of those components that are now known to be so

37

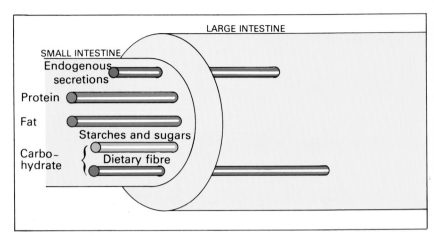

Dietary fibre reaches the large intestine almost completely intact.

important in protecting against disease. Until recently, when fibre values were given in analyses of food contents, they were related to and stated as crude fibre.

We know that fibre affects the function of the whole of the alimentary tract, although until recently most scientific attention has been centred on its effect in the large intestine, also known as the large bowel (which includes the colon and rectum).

The simplest definition of fibre – now often called 'dietary fibre' by scientists – is the part of plant food that passes through the small intestine almost completely undigested and reaches the large intestine relatively intact (above). Unlike fibre, nearly all of the starches, sugars, fats and protein eaten are digested and absorbed during their passage through the small intestine.

What happens to fibre in the body?

The accompanying diagram (opposite) shows the digestive tract and the organs through which food and later food residues pass before eventually being eliminated as faeces through the anus. The food is broken up and mixed with saliva in the mouth. From there it passes through the oesophagus (gullet) to reach the stomach. Here it is mixed with digestive juices before being squeezed by the muscles in the wall of the

The digestive system

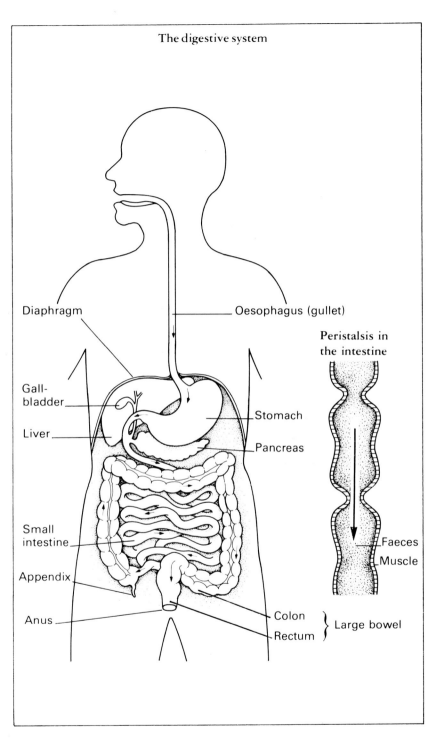

Diaphragm

Oesophagus (gullet)

Peristalsis in the intestine

Gall-bladder

Liver

Stomach

Pancreas

Small intestine

Appendix

Anus

Faeces

Muscle

Colon
Rectum } Large bowel

stomach into the small intestine. Here it is mixed with other digestive juices which break it down into simpler chemical substances that can be absorbed into the veins carrying the nutrients and energy to the liver. In the liver it is prepared for various uses in the body.

Some of the food which is not absorbed in the small intestine is fermented by bacteria in the large intestine; some of the products of this process are absorbed into the body. The rhythmic contractions of the gut or intestines, known as peristalsis are rather like the gyrating movement of an earthworm and propel the bowel content through the intestine. The bowel content is concentrated by absorption of water during its passage through the large bowel. It is fluid in nature when it enters the large bowel but is solid or semi-solid when passed as a stool or faeces. As mentioned above only fibre remains relatively intact during its passage through the small intestine so that most of it enters the large bowel to influence its behaviour in many ways.

Fibre in food provides non-calorie containing bulk. Fibre-rich foods require more chewing than do those depleted of their fibre and so put a brake on the intake of energy (see Chapter 11). Low-fibre foods leave the stomach more quickly to enter the intestine.

Fibre packages the plant foods, mainly starch, in the stomach and small intestine, which delays the absorption of energy largely in the form of glucose. This in turn controls the demands put on the pancreas, the organ which produces the insulin needed for the utilization of glucose. The significance of this will be discussed in more detail when considering the cause of diabetes.

In the small and the large intestine, fibre interacts with cholesterol and bile salts, each of which are involved in causing both gallstones and coronary heart disease, again to be discussed in later chapters.

Most of the large intestine consists of the colon. The last six inches or so is the rectum. When the undigested fibre arrives at this part of the gut, it has many important functions. First, it provides food for the growth of bacteria which are actually of benefit to the body and are not harmful. A.M. Stephen and J.H. Cummings of Cambridge, England showed in findings published in 1980 the value of this process. The faeces become much larger, that is, more bulky, and soft almost entirely due to the growth of these beneficent bacteria. At one time it was thought that fibre attracted water, but this is now considered of less importance. The smooth muscular movements of the large bowel and

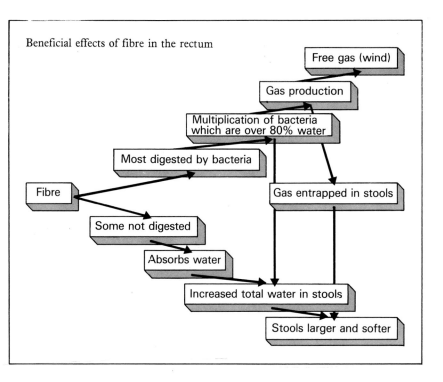

Beneficial effects of fibre in the rectum

the passage at least once a day of soft, fairly large faeces depends almost entirely on whether these bacteria get enough to eat in the form of fibre!

The liquid bowel content that enters the large intestine from the small intestine is thickened and made denser in the colon by the removal of water. Lack of fibre, and of cereal fibre in particular, is much the most important single cause of constipation, and the restoration of fibre to the diet is without doubt the most important means of combating it. Whereas in developing countries at least 2–3 oz (60–90 g) of dietary fibre enters the large bowel daily, the amount is only about ½ oz (20 g) in Western countries. If fibre intake were adequate, laxatives would seldom be required.

From this description, you can see that fibre is by no means an insignificant factor in diet. The following chapters will show in detail its special significance in relation to various common Western diseases and will explain how they could be at least partially prevented.

6 DISEASES RELATED TO BOWEL CONTENT

There are five common diseases related to constipation, that is, to the behaviour and nature of the content of the bowel. Three of these, diverticular disease, appendicitis and piles, will be discussed in this chapter and the other two, hiatus hernia and varicose veins, in the next. There is strong evidence that each is caused or aggravated by hard faecal matter, which is predominantly the result of fibre-depleted diets. You will see in this chapter how all four diseases are linked, and how fibre in the diet can provide protection against each of them.

Constipation

This common word is used to describe the slow movement of unduly firm content through the large bowel leading to the infrequent passing of small hard stools. Views on constipation vary widely. Most people expect to have a bowel motion at least once a day. Some doctors have said, quite wrongly in my opinion, that it does not matter whether you have two motions a day, or three a week.

Some idea of the magnitude of the problem of constipation in Western countries is underlined by the estimation that over £50 million are spent on laxatives annually in Britain; and over $400 million in the

Right: The average daily stool weights in different communities is directly related and the time taken for food residue to pass along the digestive tract is inversely related to fibre intake. High stool weights and low intestinal transit times are associated with low occurrence of all the diseases mentioned in this book.

Daily stool weights and intestinal transit times

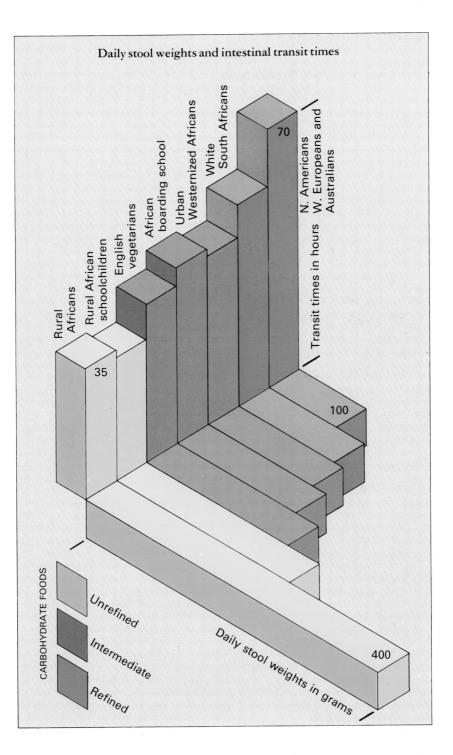

Rural Africans

Rural African schoolchildren

English vegetarians

African boarding school

Urban Westernized Africans

White South Africans

N. Americans W. Europeans and Australians

Transit times in hours

35

70

100

400

CARBOHYDRATE FOODS

Unrefined

Intermediate

Refined

Daily stool weights in grams

United States, in addition to laxatives prescribed by the medical profession.

The size and consistency of stools and the time taken for food residue to pass through the digestive tract from mouth to anus are the only reliable measurements of bowel behaviour. The amount of stool passed daily in different communities is more closely related to the frequency of the diseases described in Chapter 3 than is any other single physiological measurement. Yet there are few aspects of bodily function about which there is more ignorance. Stools are a taboo subject.

As I travel extensively, lecturing all over the world, this lack of knowledge of bowel behaviour is confirmed over and over again. One of my major research projects for a period of many years was recording information on bowel behaviour in different communities in both Third World and Western countries and endeavouring to relate it to disease patterns in these communities.

In rural Africa and other places where most of the food eaten is in the form of very large amounts of minimally processed, starchy staple carbohydrates such as cereals, legumes (like beans and peas) and root vegetables like potatoes or yams, about 11–17 oz (300–500 g) of soft stool is evacuated by an adult daily. In striking contrast, adults on modern Western diets usually pass on average 3–4 oz (80–120 g) of firm stool a day (see page 43).

The average time taken for food residue to pass along the whole of the intestinal tract has been scientifically measured and again the figures vary greatly between different communities. The people being investigated are asked to swallow unabsorbable radio-opaque plastic markers. Stools are then collected and X-rayed. The markers can be readily identified and counted. The time between the markers being swallowed and stools passed is recorded and the time taken for an agreed proportion of the markers (usually 80 per cent) to pass out in the stools can be estimated. This is known as the intestinal transit time.

This intestinal transit time averages only about one and a half days in rural communities in the Third World. In Western countries it is usually about three days in young healthy adults. Among the elderly it often is over two weeks. There is no denying that the populations of Western communities are by world standards extremely constipated. It is becoming increasingly accepted by doctors that this is mainly due to a deficiency of dietary fibre, especially that derived from cereals.

Evidence from the past

Fortunately some evidence is still available about the type of stools passed by our ancestors long before modern Western diseases became such a major scourge. Dean Jonathan Swift, the author of *Gulliver's Travels*, wrote a little book entitled *Human Ordure*, the old English word for excreta. He gave his name on the title page as 'Dr S . . . t', as if shy to disclose the identity of the author of a book on such a taboo subject. This book was published in Dublin in 1733 at the price of sixpence. In it he classified the different types of stool found in and around Dublin into five categories, just as botanists catalogue plant species. The most satisfactory stool, in his opinion, he likened to a 'boy's top reversed'. That is with the flat surface down and the point upwards. Such a stool can easily be found in Third World countries. The worst stools were likened to 'balls, buttons or bullets', an apt description of the small hard stools often passed in Western countries today.

What effect does dietary fibre have on stools?

When diets are rich in dietary fibre the stools passed are usually large in volume, pale in colour, soft in consistency and often float in water. The reverse is true of stools associated with low-fibre diets. The softness of stools characteristic of high-fibre diets is to a large extent due to the presence of emulsified gas produced by the action of bacteria on fibre. There is little evidence that drinking more water or other fluids will have any significant effect in treating constipation. Without enough fibre, fluid is simply absorbed from the bowel and excreted in the urine. Fruit and vegetables also do not help much in treating constipation.

Some knowledge of the nature of human or pre-human stools has recently been traced back to Paleolithic man. Stools estimated to have been passed over 100,000 years ago were rehydrated and their original weight estimated at about 8 oz (225 g). This is approximately the weight of each stool passed by people in rural communities in the Third World today – who usually pass two motions daily. It might therefore be reasonably assumed that our distant ancestors had bowel behaviour not dissimilar to rural Africans today, and that it is only within the last few centuries or so that Western nations have become generally constipated owing to inadequate fibre in the national diets.

Diverticular disease of the colon

In Western countries about one in ten people over the age of forty and one in three over sixty have diverticular disease, although most may be unaware of the fact. Constipation is now recognized as the underlying cause.

Diverticular disease is the development of small pouches blown out through the wall of the colon (see opposite). It was the first disease to be generally accepted throughout the medical profession as resulting from constipation and, therefore, from low-fibre diets. This is particularly remarkable as, until recently, diverticular disease had been customarily treated by specifically restricting fibre or 'roughage' in the diet. Roughage was a regrettable term since it suggested that high-fibre diets resulted in rough bowel content which was irritating the lining of the · bowel. This was a misconception, and the reverse is actually the case, so that 'softage' would have been a better designation since fibre ensures soft rather than rough bowel content. Diverticulitis, the better known term, denotes inflammation of one or more diverticula. Only occasionally do diverticula become infected. Although they usually give rise to few symptoms and remain undetected they can cause much abdominal pain and discomfort.

How diverticula develop

When the content of the colon is soft and voluminous it can easily be propelled along inside the gut by the rhythmic peristaltic waves of contraction of the muscle in the bowel wall (see page 39). When the content is firm in consistency and reduced in volume, owing to excessive absorption of water, it becomes resistant to onward propulsion and the bowel-wall muscle has to exert much additional effort to ensure its forward movement. To understand how the firmness of faeces increases the effort required for its onward propulsion, compare the ease of pushing a pat of butter through a rubber tube with the effort required to squeeze a lump of tar, or any other substance of firm consistency, through it.

To cope with these extra demands the muscle thickens in an attempt to increase its efficiency, and this inevitably results in greatly increased pressures within the bowel. In time, these unnatural pressures can force pouches of the bowel lining out through the wall of the gut. These are the diverticula (see above, right). The blowing out of diverticula can be

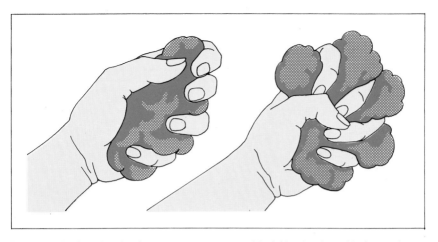

Diverticula develop in the same way as mud held in the hand is forced out between the fingers when the fist is clenched.

compared to the way the inner tube of a bicycle wheel can bulge out through a defect in the outer tyre, or the way that clay pushes out between the fingers when the hand holding it is clenched (see overleaf).

Now that the role of fibre is better understood, the idea that a low-fibre diet might benefit this disease has been abandoned. If the small, hard, drier stools associated with constipation lead to diverticula formation, then the aim must be to encourage large, soft, moist stools – a result that can be achieved by eating more fibre.

This new understanding of the nature of diverticular disease explains its rarity even in Western countries until about sixty years ago; until about 1880 the diet of Western countries contained enough fibre to protect against this disease. This also accounts for the almost total absence of the disease in Third World countries today where the daily diet is still rich in fibre.

Any treatment of diverticular disease should therefore be accompanied by a change in diet. In almost all British, and in the great majority of American clinics all patients with diverticular disease of the colon, whether with or without symptoms, are put on high-fibre diets. In some hospitals this approach has reduced the proportion of patients requiring surgical treatment by as much as 80 per cent.

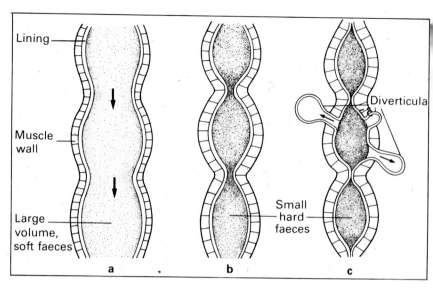

In these cross-sections through the colon:

a   On a high-fibre diet the large-volume, soft faecal content is propelled along easily.

b   On a low-fibre diet the small, hard faecal content needs extra effort from the bowel wall to ensure its onward passage, and consequently the muscles become thicker and stronger.

c   This causes increased pressures within the cavity of the gut and these can eventually force pouches of the lining through the muscle wall. These are the diverticula.

Appendicitis

I have already referred to the relationship between appendicitis and economic development, and have emphasized its rarity among tradition-ally living peoples and its sharply reduced occurrence during war-time food rationing. Appendicitis is rarely found in rural communities in the Third World. When Africans from certain colonial countries were sent to Europe for further training they became liable to develop appendicitis, which was very rare back home. In the Second World War, appendicitis began for the first time to appear among African troops who ate British Army rations.

Professor Rendle-Short showed in 1920 the rarity of appendicitis among prisoners in Britain who consumed a coarser diet than those outside. A recent study in Wales has shown that people who had consistently eaten brown or wholemeal bread had a lower risk of developing appendicitis than those who had habitually eaten white bread.

What is appendicitis?

The appendix is a blind-ended tube about 2 in (5 cm) long opening into the beginning of the large intestine, known as the caecum (see below).

Appendicitis is an inflammation of the appendix. The suffix 'itis' added to the name of any organ denotes inflammation. But in the case of appendicitis bacterial invasion is not the start of the trouble. Infection comes after the blocking of the cavity of the appendix.

What causes this blockage? How can we account for the enormous variation in the occurrence of appendicitis round the world? Why is it commoner among the young than in older people? Why does it appear to be more common during certain virus infections?

Often a small hard lump of faecal matter, about the size of a pea, is found causing the blockage (see below). This exists only in the presence of the firmer faeces that are associated with fibre-depleted diets. When

A small hard particle of faeces blocking the appendix

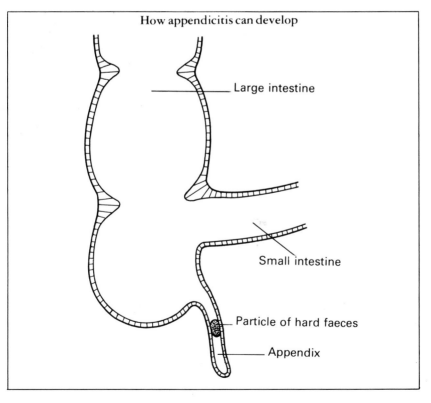

How appendicitis can develop

Large intestine

Small intestine

Particle of hard faeces

Appendix

this type of obstruction has not occurred it has been suggested that the cause may be excessive muscular contraction. This could occur through the exaggerated efforts of the muscle in the appendix wall to push out a firm faecal particle from the narrow cavity into the colon. Such muscle spasm can, in the presence of firm faecal content, close off the much wider cavity of the colon.

The changes that lead to obstruction of the inside of the appendix will depend not only on the softness or hardness of its faecal content but also on the width of its cavity. We have so far considered the former but not the latter. Until the age of about twenty, the lymphoid tissue takes up much space in the wall of the appendix, thus narrowing its cavity. After that time it decreases in amount. This lymphoid tissue swells when it becomes infected and so further narrows the free cavity inside the appendix and makes it more likely to get blocked. This could explain not only the increased frequency of appendicitis among young people, but also why appendicitis sometimes occurs after virus infections which result in swelling of the lymphoid tissue.

Once appendicitis has developed it needs urgent treatment. Although relatively mild cases may get better after treatment with antibiotic drugs, surgical removal of the appendix is usually the treatment of choice. If the patient is not seen until the disease has been present for several days the infection may have already spread beyond the appendix to form an abscess. Such an abscess may subside after treatment with antibiotics or it may require surgical drainage. In either case it is usually advised that the appendix be removed after the inflammation has subsided.

In different communities there is an inverse relationship between fibre intake and the frequency of operations for the removal of the appendix. Keeping bowel content soft seems to provide the best safeguard against the development of appendicitis. Sufficient fibre in the diet will do this. We can do nothing to alter the nature or amount of the lymphoid tissue in our appendixes to prevent them swelling up. We can alter the consistency of our bowel content by making the simple dietary changes recommended in Chapter 12.

Lack of dietary fibre is the only adequate explanation of the geographical distribution of appendicitis, given our present knowledge, and it is consistent with the clinical, pathological and epidemiological features of the disease. Here again, prevention seems to depend on diet.

Piles (haemorrhoids)

I have already mentioned that haemorrhoids, often referred to as piles, are found everywhere, though they are much more common in Western countries than among people living in the Third World. This statement, however, requires clarification, for it is only complications arising in the normal anatomical structures referred to as piles that can be considered a disease. Therefore before looking at the cause of these complications it is necessary to explain what piles are and how complications arise. True piles must be distinguished from little tender painful swellings near the anal margin referred to as 'external piles', which are clots of blood caused by the rupture of small veins under the skin. They must also be distinguished from harmless tags of skin which are a common occurrence round the anal margin.

Until recently it has always been assumed that piles are varicosities of the veins in the anal canal analogous to varicose veins in the legs, but recent research has suggested that this is not in fact the case. It now seems that piles are normal cushions full of blood vessels that surround the upper end of the anal canal to help prevent the escape of faeces (see overleaf). These cushions are present from birth. When they are swollen and are pushed down towards or through the anal canal or when they bleed or the blood in them clots they are called piles.

How piles occur

What is it that makes the anal cushions become swollen and pushes them down the anal canal? In the first place they become engorged with blood and therefore swollen as a result of the abdominal straining necessitated to evacuate firm, small stools. So long as faecal matter is soft, and straining is not necessary, the soft content comes out easily through the anal canal. When the stool is hard the straining that is necessary for its evacuation forces blood into the cushions which swell up as a result. The propulsion of a hard faecal mass along the anal canal acts like a ramrod used to clean the barrel of a rifle, and the result of oft-repeated evacuation of hard stools can be to rupture their attachments to the surround sphincter muscle (see overleaf) so that they are pushed down towards, and even through, the anal opening. Injury to the bowel lining that covers the piles can cause bleeding, and the blood in them can on occasion clot.

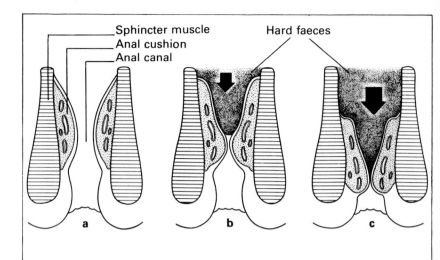

Sphincter muscle
Anal cushion
Anal canal
Hard faeces

a The anal cushions in their normal position to prevent escape of faeces.
b The passage of hard faeces forces them down.
c Eventually they can be forced out of place causing pain and other complications.

Thus one of the main causes of complications of piles is the passage of hard stools that are a result of a deficiency of fibre in the diet.

This explanation of the way piles are caused was first given by the British surgeon, Hamish Thomson, and is more closely consistent with all available evidence than any other theory. Constipation is a fundamental underlying cause. There are almost certainly other causes not yet identified, but a high proportion of patients suffering from a mild degree of piles will require little or no further treatment once they have switched to a high-fibre diet and as a result produce soft stools that can be passed with minimal straining. Many surgical clinics are now finding that, as in the case of diverticular disease, the proportion of patients with piles requiring surgical treatment is greatly reduced once their diet has been changed. Some patients will, however, require simple surgical procedures and in a few the piles will need to be surgically removed. Whatever the treatment, a diet rich in fibre is the best way to guard against recurrence of the problem.

The four diseases discussed in this chapter – constipation, diverticular disease, appendicitis and piles – are shown to have one cause in common. If they are all due in part to unnaturally firm faecal content, a very simple way to reduce their prevalence would be, quite simply, to eat more fibre. The amounts of fibre in various foods and the recommended daily intake are discussed in Chapters 12 and 13.

7 DISEASES RELATED TO ABDOMINAL STRAINING

The two diseases to be described in this chapter, hiatus hernia and varicose veins, have been attributed in part to increased pressures within the muscle walls that surround the abdomen as a result of straining to evacuate stools. Once more, the problem appears to be due to excess removal of water from the contents of the bowel, so that stools are small and hard and therefore difficult to evacuate.

Defaecation

This is the technical word for evacuating stools. The presence of firm, small-volume content in the rectum, the last portion of the intestine, has an important significance in connection with defaecation. It makes it necessary to contract forcibly the muscles of the abdominal wall to pass a stool. A resistant, unyielding mass of firm faecal matter is obviously more difficult to force through the anal canal, the name given to the back passage (the last inch or so of the intestinal tract) than a soft pliable mass. The anal canal is far narrower than the bowel above it and is surrounded by a muscle called a sphincter. When this muscle is contracted it closes the passage off in the same way that a rubber tube can be closed by tying a piece of string tightly around it. This sphincter normally remains contracted to prevent bowel content escaping, but relaxes when a stool is being passed. It can thus be compared to a tap or faucet which allows water to pass through it only when turned on.

There is another mechanism concerned with stool evacuation. Once the rectum has filled up sufficiently, the stretching of the muscle in its wall triggers a mechanism that makes this muscle contract and lets you feel you want to evacuate some stools. This contraction squeezes the faeces out of the rectum rather like the way that squeezing a tube of toothpaste forces out its contents, and at the same time the sphincter opens to let the stool pass through.

Difficulties with defaecation

The rectum has to contain about 7 oz (200 g) of stool to initiate an adequate emptying response by the muscle in its wall. On modern, Western fibre-depleted diets it is rare to have this amount of faeces in the rectum, so adequate squeezing of the muscle in the bowel wall does not occur, and consequently the muscles in the wall of the abdomen have to work more to empty the firm contents of the bowel (page 47). This straining at stool is a characteristic feature of our Western way of life.

There is another factor that may hinder the efficiency with which we empty our bowels. Throughout most of the world people squat to evacuate their bowels. This was so even in Western countries until about a century ago. In this position, the thighs are pressed against the abdominal wall and this is believed to assist stool evacuation. Modern man prefers to sit, for he knows that he will probably have to wait a long time before a stool is passed. Straining greatly raises the pressure within the abdominal cavity. Some of the results of these raised abdominal pressures will now be considered.

Hiatus hernia

This is the name given to a condition in which the top of the stomach is pushed upwards out of the abdomen and into the thoracic cavity, the part of the body above the diaphragm, which is a sheet of muscle separating the abdomen from the thorax (page 39). The thorax contains the heart and lungs, and normally the oesophagus or gullet joins the stomach just below the diaphragm.

Any upward displacement of the stomach through the hole in the diaphragm through which the oesophagus passes is known as a hiatus hernia (see overleaf). In North America this condition can be shown to be present in about one in five middle-aged adults by X-ray examination of their stomach after swallowing a radio-opaque meal containing

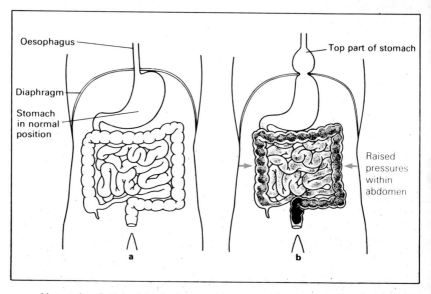

a   Normal relationship between the oesophagus, stomach and diaphragm.
b   Upward displacement of the top of the stomach through the hole in
the diaphragm that normally contains the oesophagus. This displacement, resultant in part from raised abdominal pressures, consti-
tutes a hiatus hernia.

barium. This is a material that blocks the passage of X-rays, so that when
in the stomach it defines its outline on an X-ray film. Although in the
majority of patients hiatus hernia is not associated with any symptoms it
is a common cause of heartburn. Both hiatus hernia and heartburn are
rare in Third World communities.

A protrusion of the stomach up through the diaphragm must either be
caused by a push from below, a pull up from above, or a combination of
both. The most likely cause is understandably reckoned to be a push
from below, so what is this push likely to be?

If a hole is cut in the wall of a tennis ball (opposite, above) and it is then
filled with water and squeezed, the water will be forced out through the
hole (opposite, below). The abdominal cavity can be compared to a
tennis ball. There is a hole in its wall down through which the gullet
passes to join the stomach. When the abdominal wall muscles contract
to assist the evacuation of a constipated stool, pressures within the
abdomen are increased and as a result the upper end of the stomach is
then squeezed up out of the abdomen rather like the water coming out

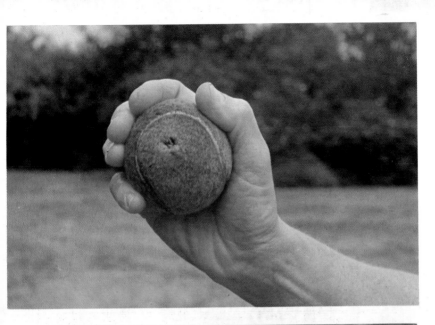

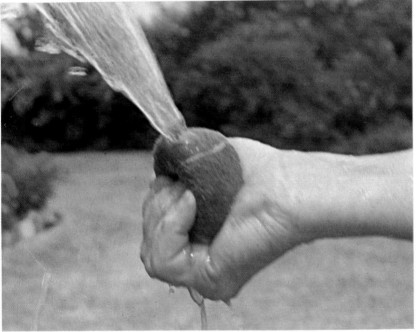

The development of a hiatus hernia can be compared to the way water can be squeezed through a hole in a tennis ball.

of a tennis ball. This is the only explanation for the cause of hiatus hernia that is consistent with the distribution of the disease, although it cannot yet be considered a proven cause.

Recent studies have shown that pressures within the abdominal cavity rise to over 75 in (190 cm) of water when straining to pass stool, whereas those in the thoracic cavity rise to only 25 in (67 cm) of water. This shows that the pressures below the diaphragm are much greater than those above. The scientists who did these studies concluded that their findings were consistent with the hypothesis that straining at stool was an important factor in the causation of hiatus hernia.

Hiatus hernia is associated not only in its geographical distribution, but also in individual patients, with both diverticular disease and gallstones. This suggests that all three diseases share some common cause. Once again, our way of life and, specifically, our fibre-depleted diet seems to be largely responsible.

Heartburn is caused by acid stomach juices entering the lower end of the gullet. When the junction between the gullet and the stomach is in its normal position below the diaphragm the muscle round the lower end of the gullet prevents the stomach contents flowing back up. When the stomach has been pushed up into the thorax the closure of the lower end of the gullet becomes less efficient, allowing acid stomach contents to enter it.

Heartburn is often treated with alkalis to neutralize the acid juices that irritate the lining of the gullet. Raising the head of the bed at night will help to minimize the entry of gastric juices into the gullet. In some patients with persistent pain, surgery is sometimes advised to repair the defect and restore the upper end of the stomach to its normal position below the diaphragm. The addition of fibre in the diet would help reduce the straining associated with hiatus hernia and might avoid the need for surgery.

Varicose veins

Veins are said to be varicose when they are tortuous and swollen. The occasional varicose veins that result from blockage of the deep leg veins by blood clots will not be considered here.

Blood from the legs is returned to the heart through the veins. To prevent blood flowing back down the legs as a result of gravity, instead of up to the heart, the veins have a series of valves which permit blood to flow towards the heart but not in the opposite direction. The flow of blood is moved along by muscle contraction around the deep veins; this contraction squeezes the veins and thus pushes the blood in one direction only (see below). The mechanism is similar to a pump forcing water uphill. The pump pushes the water up and valves prevent its return.

Veins that lie under the skin near the surface of the legs, and so have less support around them than the deeper veins which are surrounded by muscles, are more susceptible to swelling and distortion. Varicosities develop when the valves become defective so that they no longer protect the portion of the veins below them from the backward flow of blood from above (see overleaf).

Are varicose veins caused by some inherent weakness in the vein walls, or their valves? There is certainly no evidence to support this suggestion

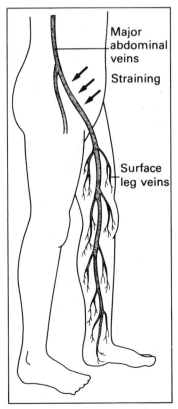

Major abdominal veins

Straining

Surface leg veins

The valves in the veins ensure that blood flows back up to the heart.

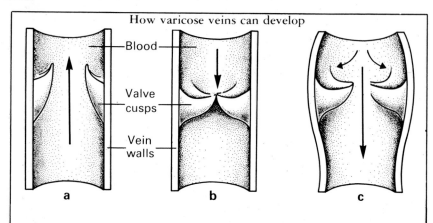

How varicose veins can develop

Blood

Valve cusps

Vein walls

a   b   c

a   The valves ensure that blood flows only back up to the heart.

b   They prevent backflow as the valve cusps meet each other and close the vein.

c   Blood forced back down the veins over a period, stretches the walls so that the valves are unable to meet.

and the fact that the frequency of varicose veins in a community is related to manner of life rather than to colour of skin indicates that they are caused more by environmental than by hereditary factors. The most likely reason why veins become incompetent is that abdominal straining forces blood back down the leg veins and stretches them. As a result the cusps of the valves can no longer meet each other and close the channel to prevent the reverse flow of blood. The unsupported weight of blood then progressively distorts the veins.

The evidence for an environmental factor
People in Western nations are affected much more by varicose veins than those in rural communities in developing countries. In Western countries varicose veins are more common among women than men, but not to the extent that hospital attendances would indicate, as women are more likely to seek treatment for cosmetic reasons. Varicose veins do not usually give rise to pain or disability.

In developing countries they are often more frequently found among men. In poorer countries with high birth rates varicose veins are far less common than in more affluent countries with much lower birth rates. These observations make it no longer possible to assume that pregnancy, or the constrictive clothing once worn by women, are primary causes of varicose veins.

Results of epidemiological studies also refute the widely held view that hereditary factors are a major cause. A survey of the extent of varicose veins among populations in the Pacific showed that they were more closely related to Western culture than to any other factor. The problem was rarest in the islands whose traditional culture had been least changed, and most common among those most influenced by the Western way of life. The occurrence of varicose veins among New Zealand Maori women is higher than among white New Zealanders. Islands with an intermediate culture, such as the Cook Islands in the Pacific, partly traditional and partly Western, have an intermediate occurrence of varicose veins.

Varicose veins are just as common today among black Americans as they are among white. In rural Africa varicose veins are relatively rare everywhere. As the ancestors of black Americans originally came from Africa this shows that the cause of their varicose veins could hardly be mainly genetic, otherwise they would still be less prone to develop in blacks. Genetic susceptibility probably does play a secondary role, but when diseases run in families it does not necessarily have to be due to hereditary factors. It could equally well be because families tend to have the same dietary and other habits.

Some people have suggested that standing all day increases the likelihood of developing varicose veins as this might place excessive pressure on the leg veins. But if this is so, why do the trishaw men mentioned on page 25 suffer more from the problem than do barbers? Only the latter are on their feet all day. The answer, surely, must be that the former are straining as they ride their modern versions of rickshaws, while the latter are merely standing still. Although the main cause of raised inter-abdominal pressures is straining to assist the evacuation of firm faecal mass from the bowel, any persistent straining activity such as trishaw riding can presumably have a similar effect.

It might be argued that all heavy physical work involves some contraction of abdominal muscles. It has, however, been shown that such an enormously strenuous exercise as weight-lifting raises pressures within the abdomen to a lesser extent than does straining at stool.

This increased abdominal pressure caused by straining to pass small firm stools has been singled out as a major cause of hiatus hernia and varicose veins. It also seems likely that varicose veins share a common cause with diverticular disease. Both diseases occur most often in the same communities, and patients with diverticular disease are more likely to have varicose veins than people without this disease. Once more, hard faeces set up a chain of events far removed from mere constipation.

Once varicose veins have developed, removing their cause will not undo the harm already done. Varicose veins often require no treatment except for cosmetic reasons. Those that do need treatment can in many cases be improved with injections of a fluid that sticks the walls together, thus blocking the cavity and preventing the backward flow of blood. More severe cases may be dealt with by ligatures that tie off the veins and so cut off the blood supply. Surgical removal of part of the diseased vein may be necessary.

Varicose veins are rare among people under the age of twenty but become progressively more common with increasing age. This suggests that the cause lies in a progressive and cumulative effect of some environmental factor operating over a long period of time. Animals do not suffer from varicose veins, which indicates that the basic cause must be something in the way of life peculiar to human beings. The evidence thus suggests that inadequate fibre in our diet is an important cause of varicose veins.

8 THE BACKGROUND TO LARGE BOWEL AND BREAST CANCER

Where large bowel cancer occurs and why

Cancer of the large bowel is another disease related to bowel behaviour and content. It is also the most serious of those so far discussed. The large bowel includes both the colon and rectum. In North America, northern Europe and Australasia it is the commonest cause of death from cancer, apart from lung cancer caused by smoking.

Tumours of the colon and of the rectum have their highest and their lowest frequencies in the same communities. The relative proportions of tumours developing in the colon and the rectum vary, however, in different communities; this suggests that some causes specifically affect either the colon or the rectum in addition to any shared cause affecting both. The frequency of large bowel cancer (also referred to as large intestine and colo-rectal cancer) is more closely related to economic development and a Western way of life than any other form of cancer.

The geographical distribution of large bowel cancer is almost identical to that of non-malignant tumours referred to as polyps. These are present in nearly 20 per cent of adults in Western countries but usually cause no trouble and remain unrecognized. Many pathologists believe, with good evidence, that most cancers of the bowel in Western countries develop from a pre-existing polyp. It must, however, be emphasized that only a very small proportion of polyps ever turn into a cancer, but the more polyps in the bowel the greater the risk that one may become malignant.

In countries where the prevalence of large bowel cancer is low, polyps

63

of the bowel are very rare; this includes most of Asia and the whole of Africa. In Africa, polyps are extremely rare. For instance, only six patients with a polyp were detected over a period of thirteen years in a South African hospital with over 2000 beds and high medical standards.

As the distribution of both polyps and malignant tumours is almost identical it is generally agreed that they have similar or closely linked causes and that these causes are almost certainly found in the food that is eaten. This does not mean that it is poisonous, or contains cancer-inducing substances, but that in the large intestine it can promote the formation of cancer-inducing substances, known as carcinogens, probably through bacterial activity.

Despite the overall size, the surface area of the membrane lining the large bowel is well over 100 times smaller than that lining the small bowel. In the latter, the lining is folded up and down like a pleated skirt, so that its total surface area is very much more extensive than is apparent when examining the inside of the bowel. This folding does not apply to the large bowel and it is why the total surface area of the small intestine is so much greater than the large intestine.

On the other hand both benign and malignant tumours occur over 100 times more frequently in the large than in the small intestine. This means that, relative to surface area, tumours are at least 10,000 times more common in the large intestine. What does this unequal distribution of tumours in the intestine suggest? Even if the lining of the large bowel is somehow more prone to tumour development, this enormous discrepancy strongly suggests that the carcinogens responsible are actually formed in the colon rather than transmitted to it through the small intestine after being swallowed in the food.

Diets that appear perfectly all right in other respects may lead to processes occurring within the gut that could increase the production, or the concentration, of carcinogens. It may take fifty or more years for cancer to occur. In order to discover what factors in diet might cause large bowel cancer, let us look at different communities which have unusually low or particularly high incidences of this disease.

Although bowel cancer is more common in richer than in poorer countries, some communities within the richer group may be less affected than the group as a whole. For example, Seventh Day Adventists, who are predominantly vegetarians and consume a diet with a higher content of fibre and a lower content of animal fat than do other

Americans, suffer from about one-third less bowel cancer. The same applies to Mormons who are not vegetarians and who have a fat intake comparable to other Americans. They do, however, appear to have a higher intake of cereal fibre on account of their greater consumption of wholemeal bread.

The life-style of Finns is similar to that of Danes. Yet Copenhagen Danes have been shown to have four times more colon cancer than rural Finns. New Yorkers also get about four times more colon cancer than rural Finns and roughly the same amount as the Danes. All these people have comparable fat intakes but the Finns eat nearly twice as much fibre, largely of cereal origin in the form of rye bread, and they pass more than twice as much stool.

Colon cancer appears to be more common in the Argentine, where a higher proportion of animal fat is eaten in the diet, than in other countries in South America. It has become more common among Eskimos who abandoned their traditional way of life and adopted an American life-style. Possible causes of these staggering differences will be discussed later in the chapter.

Changes following emigration

Many communities have increased their risk of developing bowel cancer after emigrating to another country where it is more common. As they adopt the way of life of their new country, including its diet, the disease gradually becomes just as common among the immigrants as in the population of the host country. For example, we may assume that the slaves brought to North America over 200 years ago had a frequency of bowel cancer at least as low as that of rural Africans today. Forty or fifty years ago black Americans had more of this disease than rural Africans have even today, but they were still much less affected than white Americans. Yet both groups now have approximately the same chance of suffering from this type of cancer (see page 27).

There has been a progressive increase in the liability of black Americans to develop this form of cancer as they have conformed to the pattern of life associated with modern society – particularly as they have adopted the diet and customs of white Americans. Some people might argue that this change in disease pattern might be accounted for by inter-marriage between blacks and whites but this could not explain such dramatic changes within little more than a generation. The Jews who emigrated as children from the Yemen, from North Africa and from parts of the USSR to Israel just after it had been established as a Jewish homeland, are now developing this form of cancer as commonly as other people in Israel.

The Japanese who emigrated to Hawaii and California and adopted an American way of life provide us with one of the most striking examples ever observed of changes in disease patterns following changes in dietary customs. Until the Second World War large bowel cancer was uncommon in Japan, whereas stomach cancer was more common there than anywhere else in the world. Within a generation, descendants of Japanese immigrants to the United States had a risk of developing large bowel cancer almost equal to that of other Americans. On the other hand, their risk of developing stomach cancer had fallen (see page 28).

What are the causes?

So what changes in diet can account for these contrasts in the frequency of bowel cancer?

When discussing dietary changes that follow adoption of a more Western life-style in Chapter 4, I emphasized that the proportions of calories in the diet provided by fat and carbohydrate are altered. When the amount of carbohydrate in the diet is decreased, there is a compensatory increase in the fat content, and vice versa. I showed too that fat and fibre are inversely related to one another to an even greater extent, so that diets high in fibre and low in fat are characteristic of the rural communities in the Third World among whom bowel cancer is rare. In contrast, diets high in fat and low in fibre characterize affluent Western communities in which the risk of developing bowel cancer is highest. The proportion of animal protein in the diet is usually directly related to fat and inversely related to fibre, and is consequently higher in communities with a high bowel cancer risk.

Evidence currently available strongly suggests that excessive fat in the diet increases the risk of developing large bowel cancer and that adequate fibre provides protection against it. A high content of animal protein in the diet of communities that eat a lot of meat, such as those in Argentina, has also been blamed, but the evidence is less convincing than it is for fat. Diets rich in animal protein also tend to be high in fat. It is regrettable that high-fat and low-fibre diets have been viewed as 'either-or' hypotheses in attempting to explain the cause of large bowel cancer, whereas it seems much more likely that they are 'both-and' explanations. Fat may well be a cause of, while fibre may provide protection against, bowel cancer as in the case of the other diseases being discussed.

The type and number of bacteria in the colon are influenced by the food eaten. These bacteria can act on bile salts or other ingredients of the contents of the colon and convert them into substances that are chemically very similar to known carcinogens. Fat in the diet increases the amount of bile salts found in the colon on which bacteria act. And if less fat is eaten there will be fewer bile salts to convert to carcinogens. Some of the ways in which dietary fibre is believed to afford protection against the development of large bowel cancer can be summarized as follows:

1. The production of potential carcinogens in the faeces by bacterial activity has been shown in many scientific studies to depend on the acidity or alkalinity of the gut content. There is much lower production of these substances in a more acid than in a more

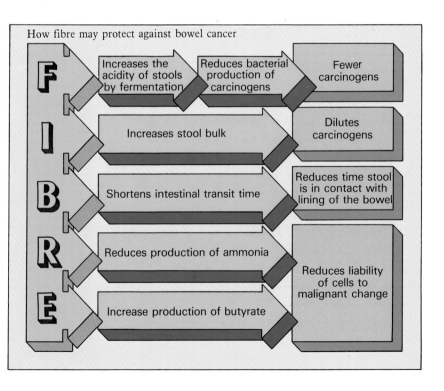

How fibre may protect against bowel cancer

F — Increases the acidity of stools by fermentation → Reduces bacterial production of carcinogens → Fewer carcinogens

I — Increases stool bulk → Dilutes carcinogens

B — Shortens intestinal transit time → Reduces time stool is in contact with lining of the bowel

R — Reduces production of ammonia → Reduces liability of cells to malignant change

E — Increase production of butyrate

alkaline bowel content. The breaking down of fibre by bacteria makes the stool more acid and this is one of the reasons why fibre is believed to reduce the amount of possible carcinogens.

2. The increased stool volume effected by increasing fibre intake dilutes any carcinogens in the gut and thereby presumably renders them less likely to induce cancer. Bowel cancer is invariably rare in communities passing large stools, and stool volume is always small in communities with a high frequency of bowel cancer.

   Research published in 1981 by Dr John Cummings and his colleagues at the Dunn Laboratories in Cambridge, England, shows that one particular component of fibre known as the pentose fraction (see page 37) – which is most abundant in cereal foods – is more closely related to both increase in stool volume and the reduced frequency of colon cancer than any other component of food.

3. Fibre also acts beneficially by reducing the intestinal transit time, that is, by hastening the onward movement of intestinal content. The time during which carcinogens formed in the gut will be in contact with the gut lining is thus reduced. This too is likely to reduce the risk of developing cancer.

4. Fibre increases the bacteria in the faeces and these require nitrogen for their growth. This in turn reduces the amount of ammonia in the large bowel – a substance that also depends on nitrogen. Dr W.J. Visek at Urbana University in Illinois has shown in animal experiments that ammonia increases the chances of cancerous change in body cells. So it seems likely that the reduction of ammonia in the large bowel may give added protection against cancer of this organ.

5. Further research in America by H.K. Hagopian and his colleagues in 1981 has demonstrated that fibre increases the fatty acid butyrate in the large bowel, which is now known to reduce the risk of malignant change.

The benefits of fibre and dangers of fat

Support for the protection provided by a high-fibre, low-fat diet is provided by the various communities described earlier. The Seventh Day Adventists eat more fibre and less fat than average Americans and have less bowel cancer. Mormons apparently eat as much fat as other

Americans but probably eat more cereal fibre as it is a common practice among them to grind their own wheat at home and then make wholemeal bread. The fibre may be protective and could help to neutralize the effect of the large amount of fat in the Mormon diet.

American slaves presumably ate a fibre-rich carbohydrate diet that was also low in fat, comparable to that of rural African villagers today. Forty or fifty years ago the diet of black Americans in the southern States was largely fibre-rich corn meal (maize) and other carbohydrates, with less fat than was available to whites. Their intake of fat and fibre was intermediate between that of Africans and white Americans. Today black and white Americans eat the same diet with the same fat and fibre content and the incidence of bowel cancer is similar for both.

The Jews in the Yemen ate much unrefined wholemeal bread and consequently had a fibre-rich diet, but after emigrating to Israel the fibre content decreased while the fat, sugar and animal protein content increased. The incidence of bowel cancer and other diseases followed suit.

The Japanese used to eat more cereals in the form of rice and millet and less fat than other industrialized nations, but their pattern of diet is changing. Those that emigrated to the United States and adopted an American way of life have increased their intake of fat and animal protein and decreased the amount of fibre they eat. As we have seen their level of bowel cancer has also increased.

All these observations about the prevalence of disease in different communities have enabled scientists to theorize as to which components of our diet may contribute to, or provide protection against, the development of large bowel cancer. As I have described earlier, experimental work has shown the manner in which fat might be detrimental and fibre beneficial. But to prove the effect of fat and fibre, or other elements of food, on the risk of developing cancer, it would need to be shown that actually altering the diet reduced or increased cancer risk. Cancer of the bowel is too rare a disease to make such a study feasible. However, polyps of the intestine (small benign growths) are several hundred times more common than cancer, and it is generally believed that they have the same causes. People who have had polyps removed are often examined annually for evidence of recurrence. Such people provide an ideal group in which to observe the effect of imposed dietary changes on the development of new polyps.

Trials of this nature are currently (1983) being conducted by Dr Robert Bruce and his colleagues in Toronto. Patients who have had polyps removed and are being watched for any sign of recurrence, have been divided into groups and fed supplements rich in fibre and low in fat, or vice versa. If those on the high-fibre, low-fat diet show a tendency to develop fewer polyps than the other patients, this could provide strong evidence that increasing the fibre and reducing the fat in Western diets could confer protection against one of the commonest forms of cancer in more affluent communities.

A summary of large bowel cancer

Diet certainly controls the pattern of bacteria in the gut, but it is still not certain which component of diet is most responsible for these changes. Various bacteria that are more common in stools from people in Western than in Third World countries have the ability to change normal bowel content, such as bile salts, into substances that could be cancer-causing.

While fat in the diet increases the amount of bile salts on which the bacteria act to produce potentially carcinogenic substances, fibre reduces this particular bacterial activity. Any carcinogens formed in the faeces will also be diluted if the faeces are of large volume; the action of carcinogens is thereby reduced. Within large-volume faeces, associated with high-fibre diets, these carcinogens will be moved along the bowel more quickly and therefore have less prolonged contact with the lining of the gut in which the cancer forms than in the case of slowly moving, small-volume faeces. Fibre also reduces the amount of ammonia and increases the level of butyrate in the large bowel – both actions helping to protect against malignancy.

The geographical distribution of large bowel cancer points strongly to changes in the pattern of diet as the cause of the disease. The critical factor seems to be a combination of low consumption of fibre and high consumption of fats. A note of warning seems appropriate here. While there is much evidence suggesting that changes in diet may be protective against certain specific forms of cancer, there is to my knowledge no such evidence that particular diets exert any significant influence on the progress of a cancer once it has developed. Similarly, while avoiding smoking will enormously reduce your risk of developing lung cancer, abandoning the habit will do nothing to arrest the cancer.

Breast cancer

The geographical distribution of breast cancer is very similar to that of large bowel cancer. It is several times commoner in economically developed than in poorer countries. It is uncommon in Japan but as with bowel cancer increased in frequency in the descendants of Japanese people who had emigrated to Hawaii or California. In America it is significantly less common in Seventh Day Adventist women, who are mostly vegetarian, than in other segments of the community. Africans develop breast cancer only about a fifth as often as black Americans, but black and white Americans are at comparable risk.

Causative factors

Breast cancer is commoner in over-nourished communities in which obesity is prevalent than in poorer populations. Within affluent societies it is commoner in fat than in thin people.

In experimental studies animals fed liberally so that they put on weight develop more breast cancer than those eating less food. Also those fed diets rich in fat are at greater risk of developing this form of cancer than those fed low-fat diets. The reasons why deposition of fat in the body and excess consumption of fat predispose to breast cancer is thought to be connected with the action of certain hormones, particularly oestrogens, which influence the development of breast tumours.

Protective factors

Important work recently presented by Dr Barry Goldin of Tufts University in Boston, and his colleagues, explains how high-fibre diets can confer protection against breast cancer. The amount of oestrogens excreted in the stools is directly related to the amount of stool passed. This in turn, as explained earlier in this book, is directly related to the fibre content of the diet. Increased elimination of oestrogens in this manner results in lower levels in the blood with resultant lower rates of breast cancer.

It must also be remembered that diets rich in starch and fibre are almost always reciprocally lower in fat and vice versa. As in the case of bowel cancer a high-fibre, low-fat diet is doubly effective, by both increasing the protective fibre and reducing the causative fat.

9 BIOCHEMICAL AND OTHER CHANGES:

CORONARY HEART DISEASE, BLOOD CLOTTING, GALLSTONES AND DUODENAL ULCERS

Coronary heart disease and gallstones – the two major diseases discussed in this chapter – seem at face value to be very different from each other, with no obvious connection between them. In fact, both diseases are linked to a substance called cholesterol. In the case of coronary heart disease cholesterol contributes to a silting-up of the arteries. It is also the main constituent of gallstones.

How fibre may protect against coronary heart disease is still uncertain. Fibre definitely reduces absorption of cholesterol in the diet, may decrease its manufacture in the liver, and increases elimination in the stools of bile acids which are derived from it. A high-fibre diet also tends to be a low-fat diet and too much animal fat is thought to increase cholesterol levels in the blood. In this chapter I shall be summarizing some of the evidence supporting the argument that fibre in the diet provides protection against both coronary heart disease and gallstones. Other protective and causative factors will also be discussed.

In addition, I shall be looking at very recent research which has shown that the occurrence of abnormal blood clotting and of duodenal ulcers may also be in some way related to lack of dietary fibre.

Coronary heart disease

This is a disease of the coronary arteries that supply blood to the heart muscle. If these arteries are severely narrowed as a result of a silting-up process insufficient blood gets to the heart muscle to enable it to work normally. This results in severe chest pain known as angina. If blood clots in one of the narrowed coronary arteries, part of the heart muscle is almost totally deprived of blood and may consequently die. This is what happens when someone has a severe heart attack. If the heart muscle is able to get some, but not enough, blood, the patient may show signs of angina or heart pain.

This silting-up and narrowing of the arteries all over the body happens gradually as we get older and is called atherosclerosis. Everyone in Western countries gets this disease to a certain extent – so much so that it has been said, with some accuracy, that a man is as old as his arteries (overleaf). Atherosclerosis often occurs first in the largest artery of all, called the aorta, that runs down the back of the chest and abdomen. Even Africans, who still get extremely little coronary heart disease, often have considerable atherosclerosis of the aorta. Among Africans atherosclerosis starts at a later age and rarely spreads to the coronary arteries. Even when it does spread the disease is less severe than it is in Western communities.

It is possible that very small blood clots often occur in our coronary arteries but that these are broken down and got rid of by the natural protective action of the blood. In Africans any blood clots are broken down more quickly than in Western people – for reasons not yet understood. Because of this and because their arteries are wider, coronary thrombosis – that is, the blocking of a coronary artery by a blood clot – is still rare in Africans, especially those living in rural areas.

Who gets coronary heart disease?

This disease is the commonest cause of death in the Western world. It is commoner among men than women. One man in four dies from it. As already mentioned, it is very rare in rural Africa or indeed wherever people work hard and have a simple, natural diet. It is certainly very rare in China except in a few large cities and is uncommon in rural India. In Indian cities, however, it may, at least in the upper social class, be almost as common as in Western countries.

There is far less coronary heart disease in the country areas of southern and eastern Europe than in northern and western Europe. Italians who had emigrated to Australia developed more coronary heart disease than those who stayed in Italy. In one town American Italians, who had retained their traditional food habits, were shown to suffer less from coronary heart disease than other Americans. Coronary heart disease increases with emigration from regions where a traditional way of life is maintained to those where a more affluent life-style is customary.

The Jews who emigrated to Israel from the then poorer Middle Eastern countries of Iraq, Iran and the Yemen had low coronary heart disease death rates on arrival in Israel. Subsequently this rate increased greatly and eventually equalled that of those born in Israel. Although uncommon in Japan, descendants of Japanese immigrants living in Hawaii and California suffer nearly as much from this disease as do other Americans. These and other examples show that environmental rather than genetic factors are primarily responsible. Undoubtedly there has been a great increase of coronary heart disease deaths in all affluent Western countries during the present century. It has in fact been truthfully called the greatest epidemic mankind has ever known.

Coronary heart disease was first clearly recognized in the 1920s after the electrocardiogram came into general use. Sir William Osler, of Baltimore in the United States and later of Oxford, England, one of the greatest physicians of all time, stated in 1920 that most doctors would see at least one patient suffering from angina during their career but that few medical students would see a case during their medical training. In the seventh edition of his classical textbook of medicine (1920) it is stated that 'Angina pectoris is a rare disease in hospitals, a case a year is about the average, even in the large metropolitan hospitals.' During the subsequent half century this disease has changed in Western countries from being a rare occurrence to being the commonest cause of death.

It has been insinuated that most of these diseases have not been recorded in Third World countries because of a lack of proper diagnostic facilities. In the 600-bed teaching hospital in which I worked in Uganda meticulous autopsies were performed on 75 per cent of all patients who died. Yet less than one case of coronary heart disease was found each year among the 98 per cent of patients who were Africans.

What are the risk factors?
There has been a great deal of research to try to establish why some individuals or communities are more prone to develop coronary heart disease than are others. In spite of much work many aspects of this disease still remain a puzzle. It has been clearly established, however,

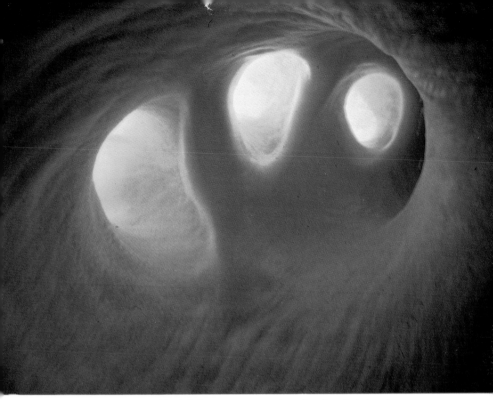

Above: This one-year-old child's coronary artery is absolutely clear.

Below: A sixty-year-old man's, silted-up by atherosclerosis.

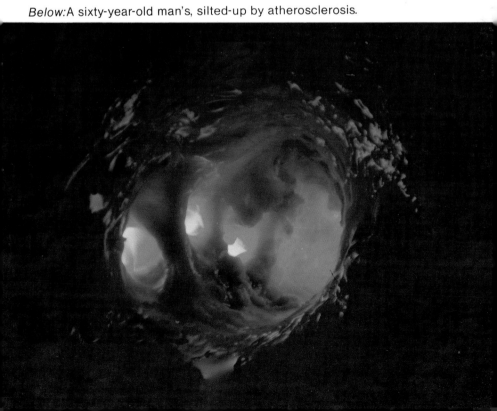

that there are certain risk factors. The most important of these are:

Smoking, particularly cigarette smoking, considerably increases the risk of developing coronary heart disease. There is, however, incomplete understanding of why heavy cigarette smoking has this effect.

Foods containing much fat, especially animal fats All countries in which the disease is common are relatively affluent and in them the level of fat consumption is high. Fat, which is present in the substance that silts up the arteries, is transported in the blood as cholesterol. In all countries in which coronary heart disease is common the blood contains high levels of cholesterol. Where the disease is rare cholesterol levels in the blood are low. While this relationship between blood cholesterol levels and the risk of coronary heart disease is true of communities, it is not necessarily true for individuals. A person who lives, say, in the United States and has a low blood cholesterol level cannot be certain he will never have a heart attack. Similarly, many men with high blood cholesterol levels never develop coronary heart disease. It is certain though that people who eat a lot of fat tend to have high blood cholesterol levels and that, if they reduce the fat in their diet, their blood cholesterol levels fall. What is not certain is whether the risk of the disease declines as the blood cholesterol levels fall. The weight of current evidence suggests that excessive intake of fat, and of animal fat in particular, increases the risk of developing coronary heart disease because of its connection with raised cholesterol levels. But it must be added that this is disputed by some authorities.

Recent work all over the world has shown that there are two types of cholesterol in our blood. One is called high-density and the other low-density. The former is beneficial and the latter harmful so it is a good thing to have more high-density and less low-density cholesterol in your blood. A diet high in fibre and low in fat makes this possible.

Salty foods Salt is considered a risk by some doctors because it may be linked with high blood pressure (called hypertension).

Certainly it is a fact that salt consumption is epidemiologically related to the worldwide distribution of high blood pressure, which significantly increases the risk of developing coronary heart disease. Inhabitants of the north island of Japan have the highest consumption of salt in the world, about 1 oz (30 g) each day, and the highest incidence of strokes from ruptured brain arteries. In contrast, communities with minimal salt intake, less than ⅛ oz (3 g) each day, such as in parts of New Guinea, have almost no high blood pressure. People living in Western countries consuming about ½ oz (15 g) of salt each day have an intermediate frequency of high blood pressure. Although in Western countries high blood pressure increases the risk of developing coronary heart disease, black south Africans, among whom high blood pressure has for many years been common, seldom develop this heart disease, so it seems as if some protective factor is safeguarding them. This may be their diet, though their high degree of physical exercise could also protect them.

Diabetes and obesity are both linked with an increased risk of developing coronary heart disease. The risk is certainly apparent among diabetic patients. This could be because diabetes itself increases the risk or, alternatively, it might be that both diseases are related because they are caused by the same common factor (see pages 85–93). A possible reason for the association between diabetes and coronary heart disease (CHD) is that the conventional treatment has been to prescribe a diet rich in fat and with a low carbohydrate content. Such a diet would be likely to increase the risk of developing CHD. Doctors in an increasing number of Western countries have stopped the old conventional treatment and treat diabetes with a diet containing little fat but much high-fibre starch carbohydrate. Fat people are more likely to develop coronary heart disease than those who are slim. This may not necessarily mean that obesity causes coronary heart disease. It may be that the two diseases are associated because they share common causes as emphasized in Chapter 1. Even overweight Africans, and there are many of them nowadays, particularly in urban areas, rarely develop coronary heart disease.

Other risk factors have been blamed. Some doctors have blamed sugar but most do not consider it a definite risk factor. Sugar consumption is very high in certain Latin American countries where coronary heart disease is still uncommon.

Stress has often been blamed as a cause of heart attack. It is, however, fallacious to reckon that stress is a prerogative of Western man and there is no good evidence that it causes the disease. Until the last few years coronary heart disease death rates have been rising almost every year in Britain, at least since the 1920s, but they fell for a few years during the Second World War when repeated bombing must have increased stress. These were the years in which imposed food rationing altered the national diet. CHD used to be most common in Britain in the social class that includes top executives and professional people. This suggested to some that stress might be a major factor. This idea is no longer accepted since the official Department of Health figures show that the disease is now more prevalent among unskilled manual labourers who as a group smoke more and are more likely to consume foods low in fibre and high in fat, fried foods in particular.

Death rates due to heart disease are now beginning to fall in North America and to level out, even beginning to fall, in Britain. This is possibly the result of a reduction in cigarette smoking and of some lowering of the intake of animal fats, and the increased consumption of cereal fibre.

What are the protective factors?

Like the scales mentioned on page 16, coronary heart disease depends on an imbalance between risk factors and protective factors. We have looked at the risk factors, and will now consider what may provide protection.

Exercise Regular and prolonged physical exercise is considered by many doctors to be a protective factor. This increases the demands of the muscles (which includes the heart) for oxygen. Consequently the arteries dilate and carry more blood to the heart and other muscles. People who exercise regularly or have to walk long distances to work may acquire protection. Exercise also increases the level of the protective 'high-density' cholesterol in the blood (page 76).

How diet can protect against heart disease There is no doubt that Third World diets are associated with a low prevalence of Western-type diseases but the reason for this is not entirely clear. Although the low consumption of fat appears to be part of the answer, few would claim that it provides the entire solution.

A United States Senate Committee (known as the McGovern Committee) took more evidence on coronary heart disease than on any other

78

disease. Its report provided guidelines for diet that included recommendations that more wholegrain foods, less animal fat and sugar and also less butter, eggs and salt should be eaten. The McGovern Committee findings will be described in greater detail in Chapter 12.

Certain types of fibre may also provide protection against coronary heart disease. For instance, when the UK Medical Research Council project researching into the cause of this disease carefully examined a group of men in London, recording their way of life and following their subsequent history for twenty years or until they died, the strongest risk factor for coronary heart disease was found to be smoking and the strongest protective factor, the intake of cereal fibre. Fruit and vegetable fibre provided no protection.

In a recent study in Holland carried out by D. Kromhout and his colleagues at Leiden – the results of which were published in late 1982 – nearly 900 middle-aged men were initially examined with regard to their health and their diet, and were subsequently observed for a period of ten years in an attempt to relate aspects of their life-style to premature death. They were divided into five groups according to the amount of fibre they consumed in their food. Those in the lowest group for fibre intake had four times the death rate from coronary heart disease and three times that from cancer as had those in the highest group. The protective effect of fibre against coronary heart disease is consistent with results previously reported following the Medical Research Council trial mentioned above. The effect on cancer deaths is difficult to understand since they were not predominantly due to large bowel and breast tumours, which are the only forms of cancer against which fibre appears to confer protection (see Chapter 8).

Dr Ristéard Mulcahy's book in this series, *Beat Heart Disease!*, provides more information about the risk of, and preventive factors for, coronary heart disease.

Blood clotting

Yet another disease that is much more frequently observed in Western than in developing countries is venous thrombosis, or clotting of the blood, which most commonly occurs in the veins of the legs. This is one of the more serious complications that can follow surgical operations or childbirth. It can cause merely pain or swelling, but rarely pieces of blood clot may become loose and travel to the lungs where they can cause severe illness or, very infrequently, death.

For nearly ten years, several surgeons in England, headed by Mr Conrad Latto, formerly Senior Surgeon at the Royal Berkshire Hospital, fed their patients with bran before and after operations, to hasten the return of normal bowel function after surgery. They were surprised to discover that in addition to the benefit on bowel function the complication of blood clots was observed much less frequently than formerly. This suggests that dietary fibre may confer a protection against this unpleasant sequel to surgery. Although these observations were made in the 1970s, the potential significance of fibre's effect on blood clotting is only now beginning to be more widely appreciated.

A recent English study on the beneficial effects of fibre in diabetes, conducted by Dr Jim Mann and colleagues in Oxford, revealed unexpectedly in 1982 that high-fibre diets affected certain aspects of the body's blood-clotting mechanisms. It may be that the number of clinically detectable blood clots is greater in Western than in Third World countries because the body's capacity to dissolve the clots before they cause damage is greater in less affluent societies.

These observations need to be confirmed but they strongly suggest that fibre may protect against blood clotting. If it could be confirmed that fibre-rich diets might reduce the risk of blood clots developing, this would help to explain why they appear to reduce cases of coronary heart disease, since one of the factors involved is the blocking of the heart arteries by clots.

Gallstones

The gall-bladder is a sac attached to the tube that carries the bile, which is formed in the liver, to the first part of the intestine. While the bile is in this pouch it loses some of its water and becomes more concentrated than it was when formed in the liver. The situation is similar to that in which bowel content loses water and becomes more concentrated during its relatively slow passage through the large intestine. The gall-bladder stores bile for the times when it is needed, that is for the digestion of fatty foods. After meals it contracts to empty its content into the duodenum where it joins the food leaving the stomach and helps in its digestion (above right).

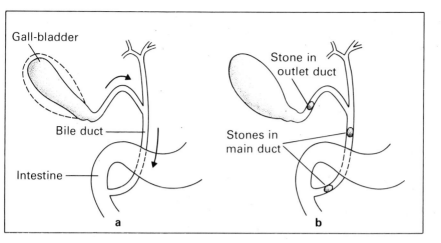

a As the gall-bladder contracts bile is sqeezed into the intestine to help digestion.

b A stone can block the outlet duct from the gall-bladder or the main duct carrying bile to the intestine.

Different types of stone can form in the gall-bladder, but by far the most common variety consists largely of cholesterol, and this is the variety that will be discussed here. Gallstones most frequently cause trouble by blocking either the duct between the gall-bladder and the main bile channel from the liver to the duodenum, or by actually blocking the main channel itself. The former causes severe pain due to the efforts of the muscles in the wall of the gall-bladder to empty its content which is blocked by the stone. The latter, main duct obstruction (right, above), is much more serious as it prevents bile leaving the liver. This can cause jaundice with all its accompanying complications. Stones can also cause disease of the wall of the gall-bladder and, very rarely, may give rise to cancer in this organ. A high percentage of people with gallstones, however, experience no trouble and the stones are commonly discovered as an incidental finding at autopsy.

The presence of gallstones can be compared to the tip of an iceberg as they are the visible sign of something much bigger out of sight. Gallstones develop in a relatively small proportion of people whose bile contains the wrong proportions of cholesterol and the solvent bile salts. This results in bile in which the cholesterol is liable to crystallize and to give rise to the formation of stones. Almost the whole population in

Western countries will have bile of a type that is more likely to give rise to gallstones than is the bile of people in developing countries.

Women are much more likely to develop gallstones than men. About one woman in eight develops gallstones in most Western countries but in some communities, such as the Swedes and the Pima Indians in the south-west of the United States, the frequency is much higher than this. The latter group, like the inhabitants of the Pacific island of Nauru (page 26), changed their diet from an ancient hunter-gatherer type to a modern American one over a shorter period of time than did white Americans, who only changed relatively slowly from the more frugal diet of the last century. Because of this the Pima Indians have probably been more severely affected than Americans as a whole who were subjected to far more gradual change. It may also be that the Amerindians are genetically more liable to develop this disease.

How gallstones develop

Gallstones form when substances in solution in the bile become crystallized. The small clumps of crystals thus formed grow in size and attract other particles to them until they form tiny stones which in time grow larger.

Any increase in concentration of a substance in solution, that can separate out as crystals, makes crystallization more likely. Decreasing their concentration will have the opposite effect. In the case of gallstones the cholesterol content of the bile is the substance that can separate out as crystals and begin the development of gallstones (facing). The most important solvents are a bile salt called chenodeoxycholate and a substance called lecithin. These decrease the concentration of cholesterol. The more cholesterol there is in the bile, the greater the tendency for gallstones to develop. The greater proportion of chenodeoxycholate and lecithin there is relative to other bile ingredients the less chance of gallstones developing.

There are other factors in the development of gallstones but this is certainly the most important. Therefore anything that increases the cholesterol relative to the solvent chenodeoxycholate will tend to lead to the development of stones and anything that changes the composition of the bile in the other direction will be protective against gallstones.

Certain components of fibre bind bile acids in the intestine so that they are eliminated in the stools rather than being reabsorbed and

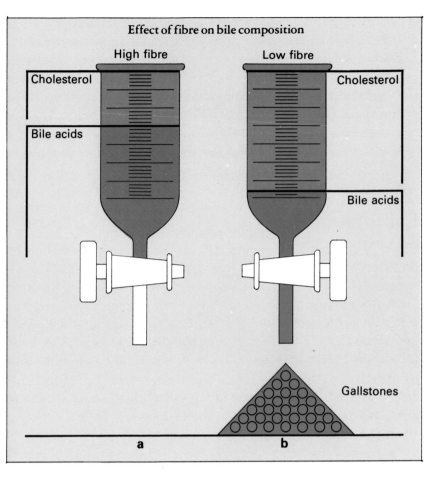

Effect of fibre on bile composition

a   Bile rich in solvent (bile acid) relative to cholesterol – no stones form.
b   High proportion cholesterol relative to solvent (bile acid) – stones form.

returned to the liver. Since bile acids are made from cholesterol the latter has to be used up to replace the loss of the former. Not only is cholesterol reduced in this manner but there is some evidence that cereal fibre reduces the manufacture of cholesterol in the liver.

Besides these changes brought about by fibre in the intestine, it has been shown that an increase of cereal fibre in the diet increases the production of chenodeoxycholate, which helps keep the bile cholesterol in solution. Gallstones are in fact commonly treated by prescribing chenodeoxycholate which has been taken from ox bile. This tends to dissolve gallstones but is not without side-effects as well as being expensive. If it can be established that an increase in fibre-rich foods could, throughout life, maintain an adequate production of chenodeoxycholate and reduce or even prevent the formation of gallstones, then recommending dietary changes would certainly be a better approach than having to remove gallstones surgically or dissolving them with medicines after they have already developed. As mentioned above, there must certainly be factors additional to diet that influence the formation of gallstones. The fact that they are much more common in women than in men suggests that hormones may play a role.

Duodenal ulcers

Ulcers in the duodenum – the first part of the small intestine (see diagram on page 39) – are a very common complaint in Western societies; but are found far less frequently in Third World communities.

A British surgeon, Mr Frank Tovey, has produced evidence that minimally processed wheat has a beneficial effect on duodenal ulcers. The active factor appears to be a fatty substance associated with the fibre rather than the fibre per se. In a 1982 study conducted by D. Rydnind and his colleagues at Oslo in Norway, recurrence of duodenal ulcers occurred in nearly twice the proportion of patients fed a low-fibre diet compared with those on a high-fibre diet.

In the next chapter the problem of diabetes is traced to diet in a more direct way. It is worth remembering that our daily diet is one of the most potent and potentially changeable elements of our environment and that over many years it can have far-reaching effects on health.

10 CAN DIABETES BE CONTROLLED WITHOUT DRUGS?

There are two varieties of diabetes, a disease characterized by the accumulation of excess sugar in the blood instead of it being burnt up as energy. When there is much of it in the blood it spills over into the urine. It was in fact the resultant sweet urine that gave the disease its name, diabetes mellitus. Fat also builds up in the blood instead of being used, and protein gets converted to sugar instead of being used for repair of damaged tissues. The common variety usually starts in middle age and is more common among people who are overweight. It can be controlled, even cured, by slimming if the person has been overweight. Adopting a suitable diet, as will be discussed below, also helps but sometimes pills that lower the blood sugar may be required, and occasionally injections of insulin are necessary.

The basic cause of the common middle-age variety of diabetes is the failure of the body to respond normally to the amount of insulin produced in the pancreas gland. Many of these patients make enough insulin and its concentration in the blood is not very low but the body is insensitive to this amount of insulin. Slimming usually makes the body more sensitive and often almost cures the disease.

The other type of diabetes, which is less common and occurs usually in children, is associated with a severe disease of the pancreas; its cells are slowly dying. Those with this variety urgently need injected insulin and are called nowadays insulin-dependent diabetics. The cause of this juvenile variety is not known. It is possibly due to a virus infection, contracted many years before, acting in people of a certain genetic type, the after-effects of which years later slowly destroy the cells in the

85

pancreas which produce insulin. These patients depend on insulin for their lives.

Only the more common variety of diabetes, that occurs usually in middle age, will be considered here. As I have said, it is treated by slimming, by diet and by pills, but a few sufferers need insulin.

Historical background

Diabetes was not unknown in ancient times but it was certainly rare. Indian physicians, at about the time of Christ, described diabetes. They wrote that patients passed sweet, sugary urine; this attracted flies, ants and other insects; even dogs licked the urine. About the same time Indian statues, which previously had depicted thin people, started to portray overweight middle-aged ones instead. No one reported sugary urine in Britain until it was clearly described by Thomas Willis in 1675. He and others considered that the disease had been very rare in ancient times. This suggests that its increase has resulted from changes in environment, most probably in the food. Diabetes is more common in certain groups of people and in certain families than in others and there is undoubtedly a hereditary element. The disease does not, however, appear until specific environmental factors, in addition to the hereditary ones, have begun to operate and somehow trigger off diabetes. It seems likely that these factors are associated with diet and changes accompanying increased affluence. French physicians as late as 1870 taught that diabetes was rarely seen in the poorer hospital patients but that it was becoming increasingly common among the wealthier ones.

Who is most likely to develop diabetes?

In Western populations a fairly large proportion of persons during middle age develop difficulty in utilizing carbohydrates (starch and sugar) in their diet. After these foods have been digested they appear as glucose, a special variety of sugar, in the blood. The blood takes glucose to all cells of the body and insulin, which is formed in the pancreas, enables the cell to utilize the sugar. This reduces the glucose circulating in the blood and the level of its concentration falls. After a meal the blood glucose level rises, then falls slowly to the level found several hours after a meal – this is called the fasting level. In diabetes the body has difficulty in utilizing glucose; the blood glucose therefore rises until eventually some sugar will leak out into the urine. The best single test for diabetes depends on the level of the glucose in the blood after several hours of fasting.

In Western populations a large proportion of persons during middle age slowly develop rising blood glucose levels even during fasting. These persons are said to have impaired glucose tolerance. If this figure goes too high they are said to have diabetes. Doctors are not agreed concerning the line that divides impaired glucose tolerance and diabetes. Most doctors consider that impaired glucose tolerance is just normal ageing and it does not require treatment because very few actually develop the disease diabetes. Diabetes is a disease; it needs treatment. On the other hand, in developing countries the fasting blood glucose level is lower at all ages than that seen in Western populations; only a few show impaired glucose tolerance in middle age and fewer develop diabetes.

Diabetes occurs more commonly in overweight persons and in middle age or old age. It occurs rarely in peasants in developing countries, especially those whose diet consists largely of lightly refined high-fibre starchy foods, little fat and less sucrose; in these communities diabetes is commoner in those who eat a Westernized diet.

Available evidence suggests that diabetes became increasingly common during the last century and the early part of the present century until it reached its present frequency and then settled down to a fairly stable level. Dr H. Emerson and Dr L.D. Larimore examined the steeply rising diabetes death rate in New York City from 1888 to 1923 before the discovery of insulin. They suggested that increased consumption of sugar might be partly responsible, as had Indian physicians 2000 years before.

In Britain diabetes mortality rates fell during the food shortage in the First World War. It has been suggested that reduced sugar consumption in wartime, compared with consumption in peacetime, might account for this. Captain T.L. Cleave and Dr G.D. Campbell also traced the rise and fall of diabetic mortality from 1905 to 1947 and related this to the rise and fall of sugar consumption.

Other authorities have suggested that decreased fat intake provided a better explanation. Dr H.C. Trowell, who assisted with the writing of this book, has pointed out the possible role of dietary fibre in protecting against diabetes. He has shown that the diabetes mortality rate in Britain fell by 54 per cent between 1941 and 1953. This fall coincided with the compulsory use of higher extraction rate flour. This contained 86 per cent of the whole wheat and a greater proportion of fibre when compared with white flour, which consists of only about 72 per cent of the whole wheat. Although sugar and fat consumption in Britain during the 1950s often rose above pre-war levels, the diabetes mortality rates went on falling during all the years of the high-fibre National Bread (1941–54).

Diabetes has hardly ever been observed in any animal living in its natural environment far away from man and feeding on its usual diet. Neither has diabetes even been described in any human hunter-food gatherer. This suggests that the disease is largely the result of a man-made environment. Further evidence for this is supplied by the observation that many patients suffering from diabetes, commencing in middle age, can be 'cured' and remain free of all signs of disease if they eat the traditional food of man, consisting mainly of large amounts of fibre-rich starch foods. Such foods would include minimally refined cereals, such as large amounts of wholemeal or rye bread, fibre-rich breakfast cereals and other fibre-rich foods which are relatively low in energy or calories. Foods such as white flour and sugar should be avoided as far as possible.

Diabetes is a very good example of a disease that is partly due to inherited factors and partly to environment. Although some individuals and some ethnic groups are much more prone to develop the disease than are others, it is only in a certain dietetic environment that the disease appears at all common. This explains both its geographical distribution and its historical emergence.

Although the proneness to develop diabetes can certainly be inherited, adherence to certain dietary patterns can probably prevent the appearance of the middle-age variety of the disease.

A good example of the influence of environment is provided by the population of the little island of Nauru in the Pacific. Its rapidly increased prosperity has already been referred to (page 27). In the early 1950s diabetes was uncommon in this community. They then made the great mistake of concluding that because of their success and technology, Western nations must know the best food to eat, and began to replace their traditional diet by food imported from Australia and New Zealand. As a result, over several years, diabetes became so common that over 40 per cent of the population over the age of twenty years are now affected.

The disease has never been produced in animals by feeding them enormous amounts of sugar and fat. Nor has any human patient ever been cured of diabetes by depriving him of all sugar or of all obvious fat. Although it has been very difficult to produce diabetes in any animal, scientists have induced it in certain small rodents: sand rats, hamsters, spring mice and gerbils, in order to study its causes. All of these animals live in dry, sandy regions where food is scanty, tough and fibrous and contains little starch.

The sand rat of the Egyptian desert has been studied by scientists more than any other rodent. When this rat is offered a completely new food, a starch-rich refined wheat cereal called chow, which has many more calories relative to its fibre than has the rat's natural diet, it starts to eat voraciously. Calorie intake doubles and soon the rat becomes so fat that it can move and mate only with difficulty. (It is called Psammonmys obesus for this reason.)

Most of these rats develop diabetes and die unless given insulin. It is not necessary to add any sugar or butter to the chow to produce obesity and diabetes – the rats' new, and to them, energy-dense food is sufficient. If other sand rats in the laboratory are fed low calorie foods, such as carrots and other vegetables which contain much more fibre in proportion to their calories, only a moderate quantity of calories are eaten. These sand rats do not become obese or develop diabetes.

The rats that developed diabetes have in fact undergone a similar change to that made by Western man when fibre-rich are exchanged for fibre-depleted starch foods and this experiment shows that such a change can result in diabetes.

As in the case of the Pima Indians, used as an example in the previous chapter, the sand rats have been subjected to a very sudden change in their diet. Similar changes in diet in Western populations usually occurred over a period of 100 or more years. It is for this reason that the increased occurrence of the disease is so much more dramatic in the sand rats which have no time to adapt to their new environment. The inhabitants of the island of Nauru also changed their diet over a period of a few years.

Diabetes has been reported very rarely in any carnivore; usually, even in captivity, they remain largely flesh-eaters and refuse to each much starch. Only about one in 800 flesh-eating cats develops the disease. All animals that develop diabetes, whether they are sand rats or old domestic dogs, are also overweight. Diabetes and obesity are somehow connected both in animals and in man and this suggests that there is some cause common to each disease.

Special diets to control diabetes

Many people who develop diabetes in middle age can be cured if they control their food intake so that they reduce their weight until it becomes normal for their height and age. If, however, they regain weight, they usually relapse. Some patients need drugs to reduce their high blood sugar levels.

It has been customary to advise diabetic patients to take little sugar and to reduce starch; this leaves a diet containing a larger proportion of fat. Recently many diabetic experts have begun to advise patients to take more starch and fibre and less fat as the basis of their special diet.

Some doctors have also started recommending more unrefined high-fibre starch foods (facing). In the United States papers have been published in medical journals reporting that a diet of unrefined high-fibre starch (constituting 60 per cent of daily calorie intake with sugar reduced to 5 per cent, fat to 20 per cent and protein left at 15 per cent) causes a remission of the disease in 85 per cent of patients. These diets contain much dietary fibre – about 2½ oz (70 g) daily.

Once the patients became free from evidence of diabetes they continued to eat a high-fibre diet. Levels of daily intake were maintained as follows: unrefined starchy foods 50 per cent, fat 30 per cent, sugar 8 per cent and protein 12 per cent.

The work has been pioneered by Dr Jim Anderson at the University of Lexington, Kentucky and at several county hospitals in England. Almost all the patients that had drugs slowly ceased to require them. Even those who had depended on small doses of insulin often found that injections were no longer necessary. This change of diet for diabetics

*Right:*These percentages of daily energy (calorie) intake from different types of food show that the diet used so successfully in the treatment of diabetes in some centres today is similar to that eaten in Western countries when diabetes was still relatively rare and also to that eaten in countries where it is still uncommon.

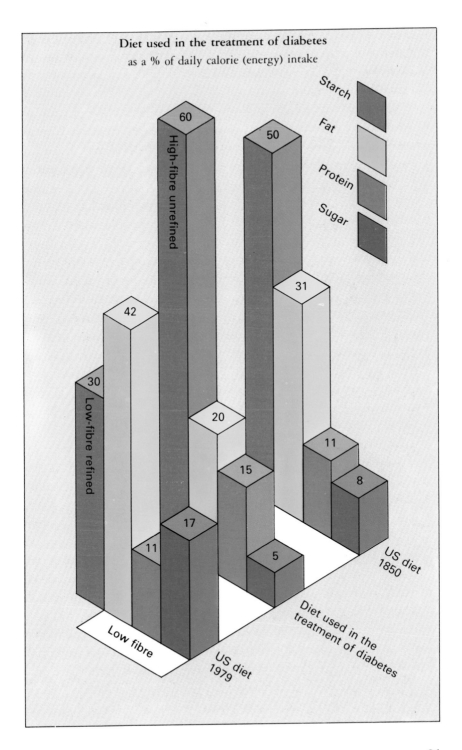

Diet used in the treatment of diabetes
as a % of daily calorie (energy) intake

Starch

Fat

Protein

Sugar

High-fibre unrefined

Low-fibre refined

Low fibre

US diet 1979

Diet used in the treatment of diabetes

US diet 1850

60 · 50 · 42 · 31 · 30 · 20 · 17 · 15 · 11 · 11 · 11 · 8 · 5

should of course be attempted only under medical supervision. In Dr Anderson's clinic patients have not relapsed after hospital discharge, while still kept on this controlled diet for over twelve months under medical observation.

No juvenile-type diabetes has yet been treated successfully using this type of diet, although recent research in Oxford, England, has shown that insulin-dependent diabetics' blood sugar levels are much better controlled on a high-starch and fibre diet than on the traditional low-carbohydrate regime.

It looks as if adult-onset type of diabetes, as well as being due to an inherited susceptibility, is most likely to appear among those who eat low-starch and low-fibre foods. It decreases, and possibly even disappears, if the diet reverts to the traditional food of Western man. This is because increasing the proportion of high-fibre starch eaten has the effect of slowing down the rate of absorption of nutrients from the intestine into the body. This reduces the need for insulin production to deal with the glucose. To achieve this it is necessary to increase the proportion of our energy needs, supplied by fibre-rich starchy foods, from the present 30 to 50 per cent or more. Average diets in Britain or North America today contain only about ¾ oz (20 g) of dietary fibre. To increase unrefined starch to 50 per cent, fat and sugar, both containing much energy but no fibre, would have to be reduced by 10 per cent.

Recent work has shown that gums, which are a constituent of certain types of fibre, increase the viscosity of the content of the small intestine, and this delays the absorption of glucose and other nutrients from the bowel into the body. The situation can be likened to watering a strip of garden. If the can has no rose the water flows out quickly and is all used up within a few yards. If, on the other hand, the water is controlled with a rose it comes out more slowly and is evenly distributed along the whole length of the garden. In like manner, when fibre-depleted diets are eaten, nutrients are absorbed quickly in the first part of the intestine. They are absorbed slowly throughout most of the small intestine when the content has been rendered more viscid by the presence of certain gums. The former situation makes much greater demands on the insulin-secreting glands than does the latter. It is interesting that doctors who have tried these new diets sometimes add bran to the diet to get the patient off the last few units of insulin or the last pill.

It is early days yet to assess the value of diets containing a high proportion of unrefined, fibre-rich starch foods in the treatment of mature-type diabetes. No patient already under treatment should change his own diet without medical advice and supervision. But no one can deny the potential provided by these findings or the practical possibilities they offer.

In Britain few doctors have found it possible to persuade patients to adopt the very large changes entailed in using the Lexington diet. However, large amounts of unrefined starch foods – wholemeal bread, brown rice, whole rye crispbreads, high-fibre breakfast cereals – as well as beans and peas, with only small amounts of fat, vegetable oils and full-cream milk are recommended nowadays at most diabetic clinics in British hospitals.

A much fuller description of diabetes and specific recommendations as to how best a patient can cope with his own disease will be found in two other books in this series: *Diabetes: A Practical New Guide to Healthy Living* by James Anderson, MD; and *The Diabetics' Diet Book: A New High-Fibre Eating Programme* by Dr Jim Mann and the Oxford Dietetic Group. Patients suffering from diabetes are strongly recommended to read both books.

11 THE DANGERS OF OBESITY

Why is it a problem?

Obesity means that a person weighs more than he should for his height and age. Medical scientists reckon it in terms of the weight-height index. During the past fifty years the weight-height index has increased in Britain and also in the United States. This means obesity has become more common in both countries. Some define obesity as being 10 per cent more than normal weight. Life insurance companies have recognized that obesity is a serious hazard to health. It carries a shorter expectation of life: for instance, if a person aged fifty years is 30 per cent above normal weight then he or she has at least a 30 per cent chance of a premature death. Overweight persons develop more diabetes, high blood pressure, heart disease, gallstones and arthritis in the weight-bearing joints; and incur greater costs and anxiety. About one-third of British men and women are more than 10 per cent above ideal weight.

Excess energy stored as fat

All food that is eaten contributes energy to the body. The energy keeps the body warm and alive; it is also spent in physical exertion. If the energy eaten, digested and absorbed in the food equals the energy lost in physical exertion and in keeping the body alive and warm, then there is perfect balance. Overweight and obesity occur if energy absorbed exceeds energy expended, since any excess is stored as fat. Most people do not have to think about how much food they should eat; they just eat until they are satisfied and remain almost the same weight throughout adult life. Some persons, however, eat just a little more food – that is, a little more energy – than they expend: they store extra fat and slowly gain weight.

The cause of obesity is still not known. But it is quite clear that overweight people do not necessarily eat more than slim people. Several experiments have estimated very carefully the energy intake of large groups of persons; the thinnest persons often eat more food, more energy, than those who are overweight and obese! Obesity usually develops very slowly over ten to thirty years. It is impossible to observe persons for many months, even years, to reckon up all the food they eat, and to estimate all the energy expended and to see how some persons take in more energy than they lose. Some marvellous mechanism normally tells us to eat just a little more, or a little less, of a wide variety of foods and keeps us in perfect, or almost perfect, energy balance for a lifetime of sixty to eighty years. Discoveries continue to be made concerning ways in which the body can protect itself against getting too thin, or getting too fat. Recently it has been found that thin persons have larger pads of brown fat under the skin, usually at the back of the body, than do fat people. After a large meal these pads of fat become warmer and 'burn off' extra energy, so that body weight does not increase. Obese persons having smaller pads of brown fat are unable to get rid of excess energy.

Obesity is certainly a serious medical disease; it is also very common. There have been thousands of experiments performed on human volunteers and on animals, who are often fattened up before being sold for human consumption, but the cause or causes of widespread obesity in women and men remains a mystery. Recently doctors, such as H.C. Trowell and K.W. Heaton in Britain and Prof T.B. Van Itallie in the United States, have pointed out that almost no attention has been paid to the role of dietary fibre in food in relation to the unsolved problem of obesity. Prof Van Itallie, who works at the Obesity Center, St Luke's Hospital, New York, has new evidence that dietary fibre:

1. decreases the absorption of energy from the intestines;
2. increases the sensation of having eaten enough;
3. promotes chewing, and slows up eating.

He also pointed out that obesity is rare among peasant populations of

Africa and Asia even when they grow enough food to satisfy hunger. Dr Heaton, working in Bristol, England, has come to similar conclusions.

Finally, obesity is certainly an inherited disorder. Inheritance is a very complex affair. In any single family some children will inherit the obesity genes, that is the tendency to develop overweight: others will not inherit them and they will remain slim throughout adult life. There must be other factors as well as inheritance that influence the development of obesity. What are they?

Obesity: a modern disease

Undoubtedly there were some fat people in the ancient civilizations of Egypt, Assyria, Rome and Greece. They were few if one can judge from the literature and the statues of those times. Even the Roman Emperors in old age were seldom depicted as being grossly fat.

The British National Portrait Gallery shows us slim kings, queens and courtiers from the thirteenth to the middle of the seventeenth century. Charles II, in the late seventeenth century, was the first man in the whole gallery to have a really fat tummy. Soon after this, in the reign of Queen Anne, nearly every lord and lady, even in their mid-thirties, was definitely obese. Before that time obesity was uncommon. History books record that in the seventeenth century the English army had 40,000 men, all of whom could march well because 'not a single soldier was fat'. Few authors used the word obese before the nineteenth century. When the word was first used it simply denoted 'having eaten' and did not allude to being fat.

Just as obesity has emerged as a common condition in Western countries over the past few centuries, it has more recently emerged in the less developed countries of Africa and in similar societies elsewhere in the Third World. In the 1920s doctors in East Africa reported that almost every African was slim. Even the soldiers who were liberally fed with traditional African food rarely appeared obese. In contrast urban Africans are commonly obese today and some of the overweight rulers are familiar figures on news media. When surgeons operate on the average African they find very little fat between the skin and muscle. In people in Western countries (and Westernized Africans) there is often several inches of subcutaneous fat round the abdomen before muscle is reached.

Africans, however, even in the past knew how to make a person fat. In the 1920s, though they bought no sugar in the shops, girls were fattened to ensure good marriage prices. Girls in some tribes were encouraged to drink lots of milk and cream, both containing fat which has a high-calorie content and no fibre, to promote obesity.

Changes in eating patterns

Scientists talk about 'energy-dense' foods meaning that they contain a lot of energy in a small amount of food. In this sense both fats and sugar are 'energy-dense' foods, the former more so; and neither contain any fibre.

Not only are many modern Western foods 'energy-dense', and consequently tend to produce obesity, but lack of physical exercise also increases the tendency to put on weight.

Sugar often provides as much as 20 per cent of the energy consumption in modern Western diets. That is, 20 per cent of the calories eaten in a day come from sugar. Fat contributes 40 per cent of the calories we eat. Since neither of these foods contains any fibre, 60 per cent of the energy eaten is devoid of fibre and is consequently a very concentrated source of calories. Fibre is the only component of our food that contains almost no calories.

About 200 years ago 70 per cent of the energy in the average British diet came from wheat and most of this was eaten in the form of high-fibre wholemeal bread. Sugar at that time contributed less than 4 per cent of energy. There is less knowledge of fat consumption at that time but it was certainly less than half the present levels, say up to 20 per cent of total energy in 1780.

Traditional African diets resemble, in the proportions of fat and carbohydrate, British diets of over 100 years ago. Modern African diets, however, contain much more fat and sugar than previously, often with the addition of white bread. Fat and sugar contain no fibre at all and white bread only a little.

Medical science has usually given its verdict thus: obesity occurs if energy in the food exceeds energy used in working the muscles and keeping the body alive. This is not a wholly correct statement. A more accurate statement is: obesity occurs if energy absorbed from the food eaten exceeds the energy used in the functions of the body. High-fibre

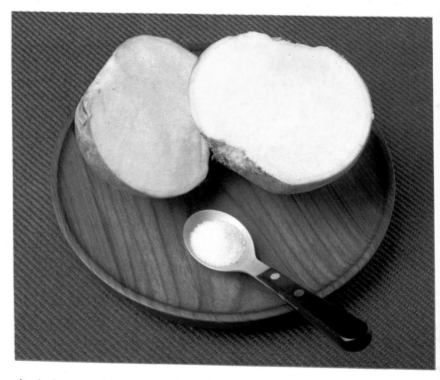

A whole sugar beet provides just one teaspoonful of refined sugar.

foods reduce not only the amount of energy consumed but also decrease absorption of energy by 1 to 2 per cent. They make you feel fuller, so you will want to eat less.

Fibre and obesity

Captain T.L. Cleave was one of the first doctors to point out that wild animals seldom get fat (except of course when they develop fat to use in winter). Neither did the average man in Europe get fat until about the eighteenth century. If an antelope gets too fat on the African grasslands a lion will catch it easily. Evolution works like that. A rabbit in Britain must remain slim or a fox will catch it. Hunter-gatherers, such as African bushmen today, or the Australian aborigines as seen by Darwin during the nineteenth century, were always slim. A fat hunter could catch few animals; an obese food-gatherer's wife could gather few nuts and seeds.

Natural selection, in evolution, is always against obesity – unless it is an advantage to survival; some fat is necessary for seals who must store fat for they feed mostly in the short Arctic summer. Zebras also must store some fat for they get little food in the dry season, but they must not get too fat or lions will catch them. Even peasant agriculturalists must not get too fat or they will be unable to engage in the hard digging and carrying necessary for their survival.

Can fibre keep you slim?

The type of obesity common in Western countries occurs when someone slowly develops an extra 14 lb (6.4 kg) of fat over fifteen years, from twenty-five until forty years old. This is 1 lb (.500 kg) per year. Food tables tell us that this can occur if only about forty extra calories are stored each day out of the daily intake of about 2000 calories. This represents only 2 per cent extra to requirements. Fibre is the only constituent in our daily diet that contains no calories. If a high-fibre diet decreases energy *absorbed* from 1 to 2 per cent it seems reasonable to assume that fibre-rich food helps to keep a person slim.

Fibre helps slimness in many other ways. You have to eat wholefoods more slowly because the food needs more chewing. This means you will probably swallow more saliva which helps to fill your stomach. The fibre is bulk-forming but still contains no calories. A person tends to eat less bulky wholemeal bread than soft white bread or cake and biscuits. Bulky high-fibre foods such as wholemeal bread, potatoes and vegetables fill you up and consequently fewer calories are consumed. Sugary drinks are soon completely absorbed, so that an hour or two later you feel empty and hungry again and look round for an extra snack to eat. Fibre also retains water, as discussed in earlier chapters. When adequate fibre is eaten both the small and the large intestine contain more watery material. When the bowels are full you do not feel so empty.

Fibre therefore both increases, and prolongs, feeling 'full-up', as explained in Chapter 5. This was demonstrated in a recently published experiment where apples were consumed in different forms. Volunteers were given equivalent amounts of apple in the form of ordinary raw apples, apple purée and apple juice (overleaf). The raw apples contained their natural skeleton of fibre; they consequently took longer to eat and satisfied hunger for a longer period of time than did apples eaten in the other two forms. The apple purée contained its fibre but it was broken down, swallowed fairly quickly and proved less satisfying. The apple

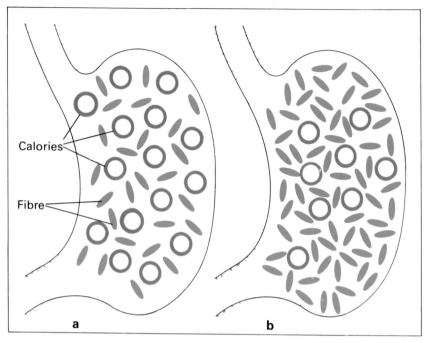

a   Stomach filled with fibre-depleted food.
b   Stomach filled to satiety with fibre-rich food.

juice which contained almost no fibre was swallowed quickly and satisfied hunger least.

Are unrefined starch foods fattening?

Contrary to generally accepted opinion it has been proved that these foods are not fattening. This is because they are rich in bulky fibre. Potatoes, for example, are not fattening provided they are neither cooked nor eaten with oil or fat. Their calorie value is in fact slightly more than apples and slightly less than pears. This was shown by an experiment involving twenty-three young Irishmen. They were persuaded to eat 2 lb (about 1 kg) of potatoes – about ten large potatoes – every day for three months. As long as they ate all the potatoes they were allowed to add as many other foods as they wanted. Actually most of the men had lost weight by the end of the three months. Eating such a large volume of potatoes fills the stomach and so prevents the consumption of other high-calorie foods.

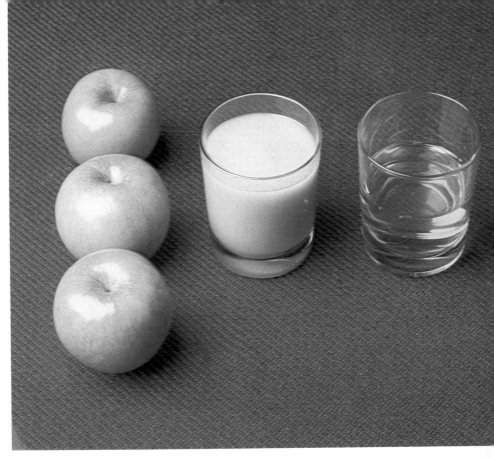

Three apples will provide this much purée or juice.

Modern medical research is beginning to study the different response of the stomach, intestines and large bowel to high-fibre diets. It is clear already that the complicated digestive glands, such as the insulin-producing pancreas, respond differently to high-fibre diets than they do to (usual) low-fibre modern diets. Scientists believe that the former diets produce a more favourable insulin response than the latter. This may explain why high-fibre diets often help middle-aged diabetics, as described in Chapter 10.

Overcoming and avoiding obesity

It is no easy thing to lose weight. If you are strong-minded you can lose several pounds, even a stone or two, over a period of several months.

But if you are not careful you may gradually regain the weight and be back to square one within a couple of years. Most of us have been taught bad eating habits from childhood. We learn to prefer foods which have a low-fibre and high-calorie content – those that look so attractive in advertisements – and contain much fat and sugar. Even after successful dieting we will often gradually return to them. Such foods include ice-cream, chocolates, sweets and cakes. In addition our tastes are geared to fat taken in large amounts of butter, cream and milk and also vegetable oils, used in frying, and salad dressing. These foods should be eaten sparingly by those with a tendency to put on weight.

It is best to try to lose weight slowly over a period of six to twelve months, and then to continue indefinitely the new food habits, rather than half-starve for a few weeks. No one can stay semi-starved for long. You do better reducing weight slowly, taking half portions of all ordinary foods that contain much fat or sugar, eating more vegetables and fruit and choosing fish or fowl rather than red meat.

There are many books about slimming and it is impossible to write fully about it here. Two points must be made. Books on slimming give long lists of foods to avoid: sugar, butter, cream, sweets, cakes, sweetened soft drinks and alcoholic drinks. As well as being high in calories these foods contain very little or no fibre, though this is rarely mentioned. The really successful slimming books are now beginning to emphasize fibre as a great protective factor. Books also give long lists of foods that may be eaten because, by themselves, they are seldom fattening. These slimming foods include vegetables, fruits, wholemeal bread, rye crispbread and so on. These foods contain much fibre.

It is difficult to prevent obesity in the modern world. People rightly enjoy eating. Both fat and sugar increase the palatability of foods. There are, however, many ways in which high-fibre foods, containing less fat and less sugar, can be made appetizing. Newer cookery books are just beginning to emphasize the importance of high-fibre foods and it is worth trying the recipes that include them. You may find, as many others have done, that wholemeal bread and other high-fibre foods have more flavour than white bread, even though at first this may not be appreciated. In the next chapter practical suggestions will be given on how to choose the best sources of fibre from readily available foods.

12 HOW CAN WE CHANGE OUR DIET?

Before considering what changes in diet should be made to help prevent the many common ailments described in this book it is pertinent to consider the relative suddenness with which we have drastically changed our diets in Western countries (see diagram below). Our ancestors were hunter-gatherers for over a million years. Then they were peasant agriculturalists, as are most of the world's populations, for some 10,000 years. The type of diet associated with modern Western culture has only

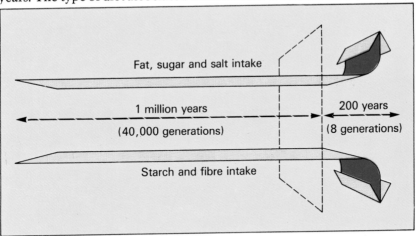

There have been more changes in the composition of our diet over approximately the last 200 years than during the whole of man's existence on earth. These changes consist of increased intake of fat, sugar and salt, and a decrease in starch and fibre intake.

been consumed for 150-200 years. We have a good idea of what hunter-gatherers ate from studies of the few remaining examples of people following this life-style. We now know that women who gathered plant foods rich in fibre provided most of the food in the majority of hunter-gatherer groups. We know a lot about the diets of peasant agriculturalists who form most of the world's populations today. The differences, however, between the diets of these two cultures were relatively small compared to the differences between the diets of peasant agriculturalists and modern Western man. When we consider what a small span of time 150–200 years or six to eight generations is compared to over a million years or over 40,000 generations, our greatly increased consumption of fat, salt and sugar, and decreased intakes of fibre and starch, occurred in but a moment of time. Any living organism, whether plant or animal, if placed in an environment to which it is not adapted, suffers. Consequently it is not surprising that Western man has had insufficient time to adapt or adjust to the new dietary environment into which he has plunged.

Once this is recognized it is obviously futile to hope for adaptation to occur, as this might take several thousands of years. The only solution therefore would appear to be that we retrace our dietary steps to the situation that prevailed before modern Western diseases became common. This does not of course imply that we return to the inadequate diets or deficient hygiene of previous centuries or that we discredit the advantages of modern food technology. The changes that need to be made vary for individuals but there are certain guidelines. There are, for a start, the dietary recommendations made by the United States Senate Select Committee on Nutrition and Human Needs to improve the health of the citizens of the USA. They are recommendations from which we can all benefit. There are also the recommendations of the 1980 report issued on the role of fibre in human nutrition by the Royal College of Physicians in Britain, who endorsed fibre as of 'great importance in human nutrition'.

A comparison of the composition of diets in communities with minimal prevalences of Western diseases with that of diets in affluent communities with maximum prevalences will help us to consider what changes would be most beneficial and yet widely acceptable. If the greatest number of people are to be encouraged to make meaningful changes in their diet some compromise has to be made between idealism and acceptability. The diagram overleaf depicts the composition of diets in Third World and Western countries and suggests basic changes that might be made. For many people starch and fibre intake could be doubled, sugar and salt on average halved, and fat reduced by a third. A further reduction in fat would be desirable but for most people not acceptable. The proportion of energy provided by protein should remain unchanged. Not only would these goals be consistent with those made by the US Select Committee on Nutrition and Human Needs, but similar recommendations have been published in the last few years in Great Britain, Canada, Australia, Norway, Sweden, Eire and France. They are unanimous in advising an increased consumption of starchy foods and fibre, and a reduction in intake of fat and sugar, and all who comment on the matter advise a reduction in salt.

Dietary goals – The US Senate Select Committee on Nutrition and Human Needs

The goals of this Committee which made recommendations in 1977 on the nutritional needs of Americans are in keeping with the suggestions already made in this book. The former advises a doubling of the proportion of calories eaten by each American in his or her daily diet from starch, carbohydrate foods, rich in fibre; it is also advised that cereal carbohydrate should have less of its fibre extracted. The Committee advised that the calorie intake from fat should be substantially reduced overall by nearly a third and sugar consumption cut by a third. Protein levels should remain unchanged.

To double the proportion of carbohydrate foods there would need to be an increased consumption of wholemeal bread, breakfast cereals, peas, beans, lentils and root vegetables like potatoes and carrots.

To achieve such a reduction of fat levels less meat and dairy products should be consumed and visible fat on meat removed before eating. Fried foods should be largely shunned. Candies, sweets, pastries and cream cakes, which are rich in both sugar and fat, should be eaten sparingly.

The American Committee also recommended a reduction of eggs, butter and cholesterol-rich foods. This was because of the assumed

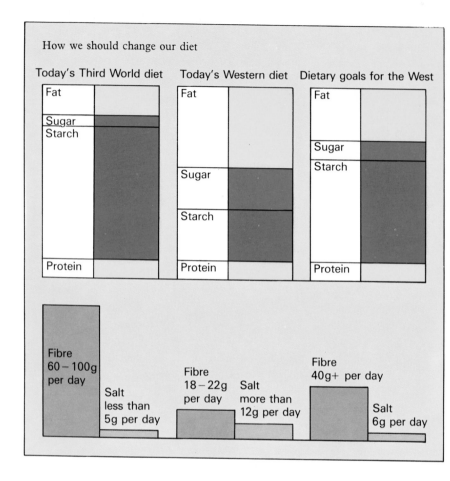

How we should change our diet

Today's Third World diet   Today's Western diet   Dietary goals for the West

Fat
Sugar
Starch

Protein

Fat

Sugar

Starch

Protein

Fat

Sugar
Starch

Protein

Fibre
60 – 100g
per day

Salt
less than
5g per day

Fibre
18 – 22g
per day

Salt
more than
12g per day

Fibre
40g+ per day

Salt
6g per day

correlation between cholesterol intake and cholesterol levels in the blood. This assumption is currently still a matter of great debate among medical scientists.

Which foods have most fibre?

So which foods should you try to eat more of to increase fibre in your diet?

The accompanying table analyses the dietary-fibre content of common foods as a percentage of their weight. The fibre content of the following types of food is given in descending order:

106

Whole cereal – (minimally refined) – wheat, rice, corn (maize), barley, rye, millet and fibre-rich breakfast cereals

Legumes – including peas, beans and lentils

Nuts and dried fruits

Root vegetables – including tubers such as potatoes, carrots, parsnips, turnips and sweet potatoes

Fruits and leafy vegetables – such as lettuce, cabbage and celery

Wheat bran (miller's bran) is rich in fibre but is not considered a food in itself. It can, however, be added to other foods.

Try to increase the proportion of food in your daily diet from among the first four groups.

The best way to increase intake of fibre-rich food is to increase bread consumption, making sure that white bread is replaced by bread made from flour that is as near as possible to wholemeal. Although wholemeal bread has three times the amount of dietary fibre compared to white bread, its effect on bowel behaviour and content is much greater than this. Weight for weight, it is eight times more effective than white bread in treating constipation and its consequences (overleaf).

Wholemeal flour contains 100 per cent of the wheat grain after removal of the husk. White flour contains a little over 70 per cent of the grain – the remainder, containing most of the fibre and much of the mineral and vitamin content, having been removed during milling. Starch is the main ingredient of white flour which, though deficient in dietary fibre, does have a useful amount of it, but not nearly as much as wholemeal flour. In view of the outright condemnation of white bread in some books on diet it must be emphasized that it is much better to obtain energy from the starch in white bread than from fat or sugar.

When buying bread look for the packs labelled 'wholemeal'. Recently many bakers have tried to avert declining sales of white bread by introducing brands of 'brown' bread, sometimes with a speckling of wheat grains on the outside. The fibre content of such loaves varies greatly and you should ask from which type of flour they were baked.

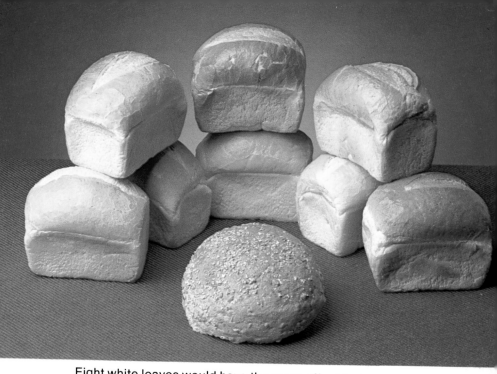

Eight white loaves would have the same effect for increasing stool output as one wholemeal.

The flour used to bake most brown breads, though less refined than white, still has much of its fibre extracted. This bread may be labelled 'wheatmeal', a term with no specific meaning, the abolition of which was recommended in the 1981 report on bread and flour by the UK Government Committee on Medical Aspects of Food Policy. The fibre content of this will be roughly halfway between wholemeal and white bread. If you buy rye bread be sure that it has been baked with unrefined rye flour. Bakers often bake so-called 'rye' bread with refined rye flour, merely adding some rye seeds to it. The report I referred to above strongly recommended, as a result of a two-year inquiry, not only that bread should provide more of our nutritional needs but also that a greater proportion of it should be brown or wholemeal. It also recommended that the extraction rate or the fibre content of bread should be indicated on the wrapping – a practice that has been adopted by a number of the major bread-producing companies.

Our ancestors ate about 1¼ lb (over 600 g) of bread, made from little-processed flour, per person per day. Current intake in Western countries is usually only about ¼ lb (120 g) of white bread. Between ¼ and ½ lb (120–240 g) of wholemeal bread daily would be adequate to supply most of the fibre necessary to combat constipation. Fibre from other sources besides bread would also be required.

The value of bran

Another good way of meeting fibre requirements is from fibre-rich breakfast cereals. There are many varieties on the market. All those containing the word 'bran', and several others besides, are good sources of fibre.

The richest of all sources of cereal fibre is wheat bran composed of the outer layers of the wheat which are removed in the preparation of white flour (page 37). This can be bought as miller's bran. Try to get the fairly coarse flakes, rather than fine, as they are more effective. Two heaped dessertspoonfuls (tablespoons in the US) a day provide about ½ oz (15 g)

One heaped tablespoonful of bran eaten daily is usually sufficient to combat constipation.

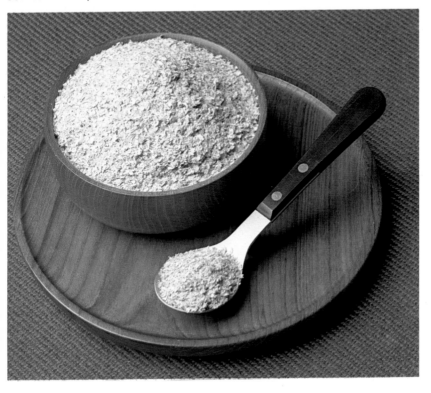

of bran containing ¼ oz (7 g) of dietary fibre. This is more than enough for most people to revolutionize beneficially their bowel behaviour. When starting to take bran, it is best to commence slowly with half the amounts suggested, to reduce wind, and then increase gradually.

Vegetables and fruit

Legumes, that is, peas, beans, and lentils, are the next best source of fibre after cereals. There is 1 oz (30 g) of dietary fibre in 9 oz (280 g) of frozen peas and a little more in the same weight of canned baked beans.

Root vegetables, including tubers like potatoes and carrots, can provide an adequate fibre intake. Considerable quantities have to be eaten, however. Potatoes baked in their skins have a higher fibre content than boiled, peeled potatoes. Although some vitamins are lost in the actual boiling of these and other vegetables, our bodies have become adjusted over innumerable generations to eating cooked food. Indeed it is difficult to eat starch unless it is cooked first.

The main thing to remember when eating potatoes is to avoid having them fried which adds a high concentration of fat and trebles their calorie content. As mentioned earlier, potatoes are not fattening unless cooked in fat or eaten with butter or cream. Incredible though it may seem, during the nineteenth century farm labourers in Ireland lived on one pint of milk and ten pounds of potatoes a day. Although this diet can hardly be considered ideal, it apparently fulfilled their nutritional needs. Fresh fruit and vegetables contain fibre but they are composed largely of water. In the case of salads, for instance, it clearly would not be possible to eat anywhere near the quantity that would be required to meet our fibre requirements. There has been a trend to eat more salad, consisting largely of lettuce, heavily soaked in salad dressing containing fat. Prof Peter Van Soest – one of the greatest fibre experts in North America – has stated that 'salad is little more than packaged water'. Spinach does have a relatively high fibre level, as you can see from the table on page 120.

An overall change in diet

Reduction in consumption of fatty foods, especially animal fats, implies a reduced intake of meat and, in particular, of red meat such as beef, lamb and pork. Animals providing these meats have been specifically

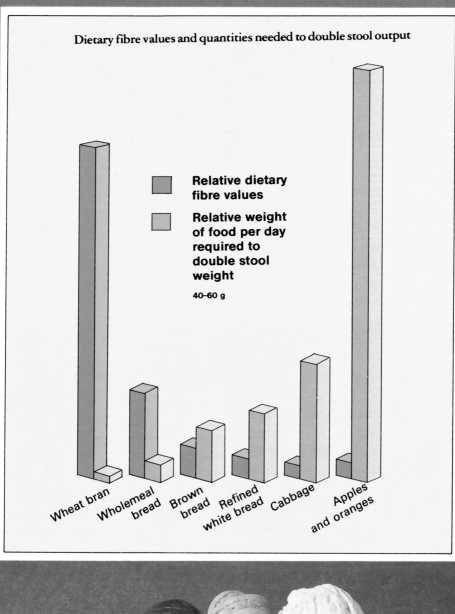

Dietary fibre values and quantities needed to double stool output

Relative dietary fibre values

Relative weight of food per day required to double stool weight

40–60 g

Wheat bran

Wholemeal bread

Brown bread

Refined white bread

Cabbage

Apples and oranges

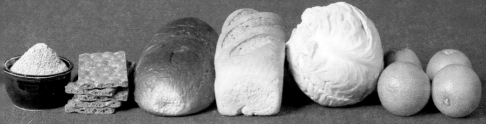

bred to increase the fat in their carcasses. Try to eat leaner meats instead of fatty ones. White meats, such as fish and poultry, have a much lower fat content, but duck and goose can be rich in fat.

Consumption of refined carbohydrate foods, of which sugar is the most obvious example, should be reduced. We need to cut sugar to half or less of our present consumption of about 100 lb (45 kg) per person per year. The photograph on page 98 gives an idea of the amount of sugar beet that would have to be eaten to consume the energy contained in a teaspoonful of sugar. So eat fewer sweetened foods and drink less cola and other soft drinks which contain about 10 per cent sugar by weight. Foods composed largely of sugar and white flour should be consumed sparingly though it would be quite impractical and unacceptable to suggest that they should be entirely excluded from our diet.

Points about bran

As a treatment for constipation bran has been found to be most effective, though popular fibre-rich breakfast cereals are also helpful as they are more palatable. Bran from health food shops and many supermarkets, can be added to dry breakfast cereals or oatmeal porridge, sprinkled on stewed fruits, mixed into soups or added to the flour when preparing home-made bread. When making bread add 1–2 oz (30–60 g) to 1 lb (500 g) of flour.

Start with one heaped teaspoonful a day, increasing by one heaped teaspoon after the first week. Then increase gradually as needed till at least one soft stool is passed daily, and keep to this daily amount. You may experience wind for several weeks while you are new to bran, but eventually this will largely disappear. It is possible to obtain bran tablets or other concentrated-fibre products. These are useful for holidays and times spent away from home when fibre-rich meals may not be available, but even for these occasions an increasing number of people carry their bran with them.

Practical hints – what to eat, what to avoid

During the few years since this book was first published, I have repeatedly been asked for suggestions on how to include fibre in an ordinary, everyday diet. I have therefore decided to add a section with practical guidelines that I hope you will find useful.

A considerable amount of confusion on this subject is caused by a small group of people who advise such absolutes when talking about food that much of their advice is difficult to follow and consequently quite unacceptable to most of us. I have heard it suggested, for instance, that every item of food containing any sugar or white flour must at all costs be avoided. But who could possibly go to a wedding reception and refuse the wedding cake! The important thing is to learn how to eat sensibly most of the time, so that when you come to having a day or evening out, you can happily relax and enjoy yourself.

The basic principles of eating which I am going to recommend here embody the large mass of current, informed medical opinion and are not merely the views of any one individual. In particular, I will endeavour to underline the fundamental points to follow and to emphasize the importance of the correct allocation of priorities. In any action taken, you must find the balance between the advantages gained and the risks accepted – and if the advantages hugely outweigh the risks, then surely the action is worth taking.

In my experience, most diets tell us what not to do rather than concentrating on the more positive aspects. The emphasis always seems to be avoid, avoid, avoid! Conversely, my emphasis throughout this book has been that a diet rich in starch and fibre, and low in fat and sugar *protects* against disease and is at the same time nourishing, filling and enjoyable to eat.

Fibre-rich foods, as we have seen, are foods such as wholemeal bread, fibre-rich breakfast cereals, wholemeal pasta, peas, beans, lentils and root vegetables, such as potatoes, turnips, parsnips and carrots. Basically, you should try to eat more of these foods and far less fat, and in particular animal fat.

Breakfast
The best meal to focus your fibre intake on is breakfast for the following reasons:

- It is the easiest meal to control because it is usually eaten at home.
- Cereal foods are high in fibre and breakfast is the meal that lends itself *par excellence* to a predominantly cereal meal.
- One of the best ways to supplement your diet with fibre is with bran – simply by adding two dessertspoonfuls (tablespoonfuls in America)

of bran to your morning cereal. (Bran can also be used in many other ways, such as for thickening soups, sauces and even hot-pots.)

By the word 'cereal', I am referring to anything which is botanically a cereal, in other words, wheat, maize, oats and even wholemeal bread, which is made from the whole grain of wheat. It is always better to eat somewhere near wholemeal bread (100 per cent extraction) or other high-fibre breads (over 80 per cent) instead of white bread.

If you can manage to have a breakfast based on a high-fibre packet cereal, oatmeal porridge with added bran, muesli or wholemeal bread, cutting down on cooked breakfasts, you immediately have an excellent high-fibre meal. If you're used to eating a hefty breakfast, don't be afraid to take a good plateful of cereal – even a soup-bowl size – and not an amount that is so small that you will feel hungry almost as soon as you've eaten it. You'll soon find that a good cereal breakfast will not only fill you up, but will keep you going for many hours.

At the same time, make sure that you enjoy your cereal. Don't worry if you prefer to eat it with a little sugar or sweetener. The amounts we are talking about are really very small.

The same applies to milk. It is far better to have cereal with milk (even if it does contain some fat) than not to have any cereal at all. The essential thing is to get your priorities right. A bowl of dry cereal would be difficult to eat! If you are really concerned and wish to lose weight, try using skimmed milk, from which most of the fat has been removed.

Again, with wholemeal bread, better to have a little margarine or marmalade with it if that's how you enjoy it, rather than not have it at all. The amount of sugar contained in marmalade is immaterial, compared to the amount of sugar people include in drinks such as tea or coffee – and the fat in the margarine is nothing compared to the fat in a piece of meat!

Tea drinking is another area where there often seems to be confusion: the dangers or hazards attributed to tea drinking are largely hypothetical. It is vastly more important to have a substantial breakfast, accompanied by a cup of tea or coffee, than to dash out and simply have a cup of coffee and a sweet bun during the morning.

In North America, and increasingly in Britain, it is becoming much more common to have a glass of fruit juice with your breakfast, rather than to eat a whole piece of fruit – yet the fruit itself is much better for us. The fibre in the fruit is very valuable and we really don't need the juice alone, as we are short of neither water nor vitamins. In fact, from a purely health point of view, we would be better off to eat the fibre than drink the juice.

The final reason for a cereal-based breakfast is that we should all avoid fried food, except on special occasions. The amount of fat present in such foods can be as detrimental as fibre is beneficial.

● Bacon should be eaten sparingly because we all eat too much salt. Smoked meats and fish also have a high salt content.

● Sausages have almost the highest fat content of any food.

● Eggs need not be discarded but should be eaten in moderation. There is a difference of opinion among nutritionists as to the relative benefits or dangers of eating eggs. They are a very rich source of cholesterol.

The fried breakfast served with white toast – the meal that is still provided in almost every hotel – is the one meal that is contrary to all that this book recommends.

The main meal of the day

For the purposes of this book, I will assume that the main meal of the day is taken in the evening, but the advice given here can of course be switched round to a midday meal.

Like breakfast, this meal is very often taken at home and is therefore easier to control. Normally it is made up of meat, potatoes and other vegetables and perhaps a dessert.

The fundamental change I would suggest here is to increase the proportions of vegetables, and particularly potatoes, relative to the meat. So instead of having a meat-based meal supplemented with vegetables, it would be much better if you could get used to having a vegetable-based meal supplemented with meat. As William Connor, the well-known American nutritionist, has pointed out, 'The time will come, primarily due to economic pressures, when meat will be used as a condiment to flavour other foods.'

Here are some practical hints to follow:

● Eat meat no more than once a day and, when you do, eat it sparingly. About 4 oz (120 g) is quite sufficient for an adult.

- Cut the fatty parts out of meat. The leanest meats are chicken and turkey (better to discard the skin).
- Fish other than mackerel, salmon and sardines is less fatty and has fewer calories than meat, weight for weight.
- Grill (broil) instead of fry. Use nonstick pans or skillets for frying with minimum fat.
- Potatoes can be eaten freely – provided they are not cooked or eaten with fat. It is also preferable to eat them with their skins left on.
- Salads provide a pleasant accompaniment to meals but are *not* high in fibre. Avoid a large amount of high-fat dressing.
- Peas, beans, lentils and brown rice are all high in fibre and provide excellent accompaniments to the main dish. They are also filling, so you will find that when they are served you will be quite happy to eat less meat or fish than you are accustomed to.
- Peas, beans, lentils and brown rice can all provide delicious, inexpensive main dishes in their own right, from wonderful warming soups to all sorts of tasty hot-pots.

Snack meals

Your third meal of the day – whether at midday or in the evening – need only be a light snack. I would advise you to keep between-meal snacks to a minimum. At home, my wife and I almost always have a lunch based on wholemeal bread, and with it we usually eat a little margarine, yeast extract, cheese, honey or marmalade. High-fibre foods, however, lend themselves very well to snack meals and a few other suggestions are:

- A pasta snack, such as spaghetti or macaroni, using wholemeal pasta.
- A snack made with brown rice, such as a rice salad. (Brown, rice takes longer to cook than white rice, approximately ¾ hour.)
- Baked beans on a piece of wholemeal toast.
- A pizza made with wholemeal flour.
- A fibre-rich vegetable soup with wholemeal bread.
- A salad made with nuts or dried fruits.
- Sandwiches made with wholemeal bread – try to have more bread and less filling in each one.

Desserts

This is a more difficult area to advise on. The more exotic ones should be kept for weekends and special occasions. Often, at home, we end our

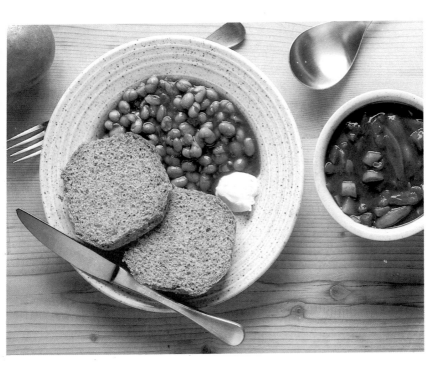

meal with a piece of fruit, rather than a dessert. Fruit salads, fruit pies, baked apples, stuffed with nuts and raisins and compôtes made with dried fruits all make pleasant fruit desserts.

- When possible eat fresh rather than canned fruit. The latter usually has a high sugar content. Avoid fruits canned with heavy syrup, which is laden with sugar.
- Use butter sparingly. Add less cream to desserts and reduce sugar as much as possible.
- Brown sugar has no health advantages over white. Both are termed 'empty calories' as they provide energy but virtually nothing else.
- Substitute a high-extraction (80–100 per cent) flour for white in homemade pastries and piecrust, cakes, biscuits (cookies), and bread.
- Bran and All-Bran or similar products can be used to make delicious crunchy toppings for fruit crumbles.

If you want to find out more about high-fibre cookery along the lines I have suggested above, I thoroughly recommend *The High-Fibre Cookbook: Recipes For Good Health*, by Pamela Westland, also in this series.

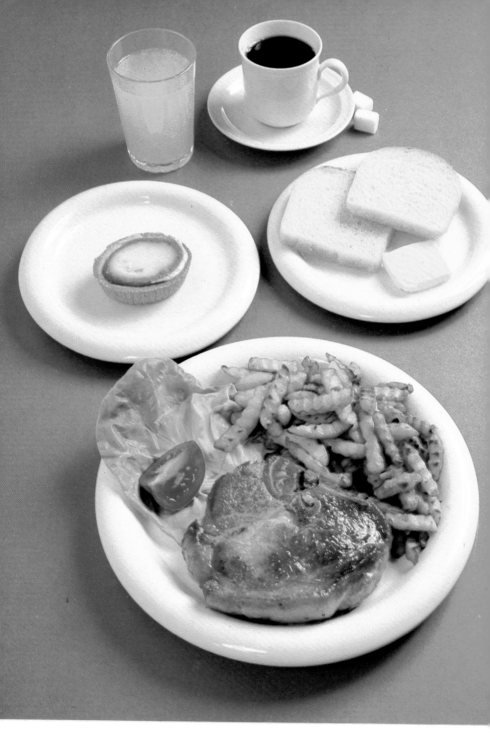

Above: This meal contains minimal fibre but too much fat and sugar.

Right: Most of the food shown here is rich in fibre while containing little fat and no added sugar.

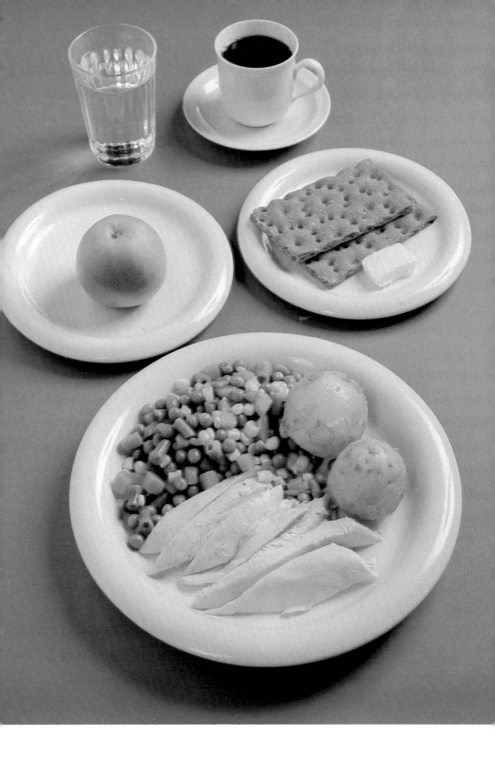

Dietary fibre values of food
Expressed as a percentage by weight (per 100 grams)

Cereals	%
Wheat bran (miller's bran)	44.0
Wholemeal flour (100% unrefined)	9.6
Brown flour (85% refined)	7.5
White flour (72% refined)	3.0
Soya flour (low fat)	14.3
Sweetcorn, canned	5.7
Corn-on-the-cob, boiled	4.7
Rice, white polished, boiled	0.8
brown, unpolished, boiled	5.5

Bread	
Wholemeal	8.5
Brown	5.1
Hovis (UK)	4.6
White	2.7

Breakfast cereals	
All-Bran	28.3
Bran Buds	26.2
Puffed Wheat	15.4
Bran Flakes	14.7
Sultana Bran	12.8
Weetabix	12.7
Shredded Wheat	12.3
Muesli	7.4
Grapenuts	7.0
Sugar Puffs	6.1
Country Store	5.1
Cornflakes	2.0
Special K	1.6
Rice Krispies	1.0
Porridge	0.8

Biscuits	
Ry-King Fibre Plus	28.0
Crispbread rye (Ryvita)	11.7
Digestive, plain	5.5
Energen crispbread	4.9
Shortbread	2.1

Nuts	
Almonds	14.3
Coconut, fresh	13.6
Brazil	9.0
Peanuts	8.1
Hazel	6.1

Vegetables	
Spinach, boiled	6.3
Spring greens, boiled	3.8
Spring onions	3.1
Broccoli tops, boiled	2.9
Brussel sprouts, boiled	2.9
Aubergines, raw	2.5
Cabbage, boiled	1.8
Cauliflower, boiled	1.8
Celery, raw	1.8
Lettuce	1.5
Onions, boiled	1.3
Asparagus, cooked	0.8
Marrow, boiled	0.6
Cucumber, raw	0.4

Root vegetables	
Horseradish, raw	8.3
Kidney beans, cooked	7.4
Butter beans, cooked	5.1
Yam, boiled	3.9
Carrots, boiled	3.0
raw	2.9
Parsnips, boiled	2.5
Beetroots, boiled	2.5
Potatoes, baked in skins (flesh only)	2.5
Turnip, boiled	2.2
Potatoes, boiled (new)	2.0

Legumes	
Peas, frozen, boiled	12.0
Beans, haricot (whole beans), boiled	7.4
baked and canned in tomato sauce	7.3
Peas, canned	6.3
fresh, boiled	5.2
Broad beans, boiled	5.1
Lentils, split, boiled	3.7
Runner beans, boiled	3.4

Fruits	
Dates, dried	8.7
Prunes, stewed	7.4
Raspberries	7.4
Blackberries	7.3
Raisins	6.8
Cranberries	4.2
Bananas	3.4
Pears, fresh, eating	3.3
Strawberries	2.2
Plums, raw, eating	2.1
Apples	2.0
Oranges	2.0
Cherries	1.7
Apricots, stewed	1.6
Tomatoes, raw	1.5
Peaches	1.4
Pineapple, fresh	1.2
Grapes	0.9
Melon (honeydew)	0.9
Grapefruit	0.6

Puddings	
Apple crumble	2.5
Fruit pie	2.4
Rhubarb, stewed – no sugar	2.4
Christmas pudding	2.0
Sponge	1.2

13 NOT BY BREAD ALONE

Prevention, as we all know, is far preferable to cure. It is often more of an effort to achieve, however, because it involves changing people's habits and attitudes.

Most modern medicine is concentrated on cure rather than on prevention. It can be compared to stationing an ambulance at the foot of a cliff to pick up the casualties as men and women fall over and sustain injuries of various kinds. The efficient ambulance takes the patients to medical centres equipped with all modern facilities and staffed with highly trained medical teams. This is important and necessary work. But how much better it would be to erect a fence around the top of the cliff to prevent people from falling off in the first place! Giving up cigarette smoking, moderation in alcohol, and eating a prudent diet are all examples of ways we can build fences around our cliffs and so avoid many preventable diseases.

An even more telling illustration is that of a running tap filling a basin from which the overflow is flooding the floor. Two men work long hours mopping up the water, their aim in life being to keep the floor dry (overleaf). Yet it has never occurred to them that turning off the tap would enormously reduce the need to mop the flooded floor. The running water represents the cause of disease and the flood on the floor the diseases filling hospital beds and doctors' surgeries.

A medical student learns the standard techniques of floor-mopping but has minimal instruction in finding and turning off running taps or, in other words, in discovering and eradicating the causes of disease. Industrial enterprises provide the best mops man's ingenuity can devise

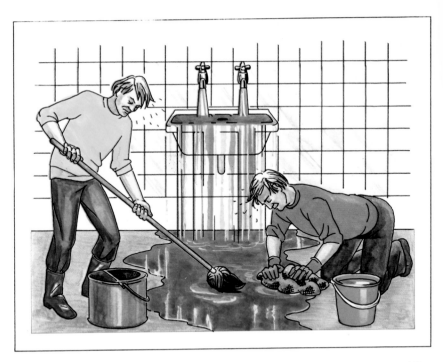

These two men are fruitlessly mopping up the overflowing water while omitting to turn off the tap or faucet.

in the form of pharmaceutical preparations, surgical appliances and laboratory technology. For all of these we must be grateful, but let them not blind us to the need to search for and eradicate causes of disease at their source.

The analogy is plain. There is, and always will be, a flood on the floor, the presence of disease in the world, which must be dealt with by the best means possible. But how much better it would be to turn off the tap as well as mopping the floor, rather than ignoring the former while concentrating on the latter. I myself spent five years as a medical student learning to diagnose and treat disease. I learnt little about preventive medicine, and almost nothing about diet. After qualifying I studied for higher diplomas, learning more advanced techniques in floor-mopping. Not until after nearly thirty years of what I believe to be important floor-mopping in the form of surgery did I begin to realize the paramount importance of looking for and endeavouring to turn off taps.

You could say, in the face of the ideas presented in this book, that we do not yet have sufficient proof concerning the turning off of this particular tap – fibre-depleted diets. But to use another example, if a man has fallen into the water and there is a lifebelt at hand you throw it to him. You would hardly ponder whether it is the right size, the correct shape or specific gravity while the man meanwhile drowns! The testing can be done subsequently so as to improve rescue arrangements for future needs. There is still much testing to be done regarding diet but meanwhile we do have sufficient knowledge on which we can act and also sufficient knowledge to say that, if Third World communities adopt our kind of diet, they do so at their peril.

Beyond biological reckoning

It might well be argued – and I fully agree – that the welfare of individuals is only partially ensured by caring for their biological needs. Were a human being no more than a chemical factory, or even a purely biological creature, the adequate meeting of bodily needs alone would provide satisfaction and fulfilment, yet it is patently obvious that this is far from the case. I have endeavoured to show in this book that, from a dietary point of view, we have concentrated on the content of plant cells, the nutrients they contain and ignored the carton, the cell wall, the undigested fibre. It is all too easy when dealing with patients to concentrate so much on the carton, man's biological body, that we ignore the content, man himself as a person. Lord Tennyson wrote, 'I am not my skeleton and consequently I am not greatly concerned where my skeleton came from.' Some 5000 years before Tennyson it was written in the book of Deuteronomy 8: 3 that: 'Man cannot live by bread alone', bread referring not only to food, an essential requirement for life, as discussed in this book, but representing all the needs of our biological natures. The quote continues, 'but by every word that God utters', implying that man is something more than a merely biological creature.

In recent years there has been an increasing appreciation of the essential inter-relationship between mind and body in the maintenance of health. The Greeks used the word 'soma' to denote the body and 'psyche' to describe the mind. The term psychosomatic disease implies illness explicable in part by purely physical changes but in which other factors such as anxiety, insecurity or the tensions of a stressful relationship also play a part. Many doctors widen this concept even further to include the component of man's nature for which the Greeks used the word 'pneuma', referring to man's true self or spirit, that additional dimension which would seem to differentiate man from all other animals.

A book on the relationship between food and health must inevitably emphasize biological or body disease almost to the exclusion of other aspects of well-being. I am anxious that this should in no way detract from the truth that man is an entity comprising body, mind and spirit, an order of priorities which should be reversed in conformity with Tennyson's comment referred to above, or with St Paul's prayer for his Thessalonian friends that they be kept in spirit, mind and body (I Thessalonians 5: 23).

The basic concept of health is that of wholeness. This involves every component of man's being and also inter-relationships with one another. We have in our own hands the means to improve the nourishment, and consequently the health and fulfilment, of all three components of our nature. In respect of the purely biological there is far too great a tendency to resort to drugs rather than recognizing and avoiding the causes of disease. I hope this book will help to overcome this tendency.

ACKNOWLEDGEMENTS

I want to thank my wife, Olive. Her support and help have been invaluable, not least on the many occasions when my work has taken me away from my happy home.

I am greatly indebted to Dr Hugh Trowell, former Senior Consultant Physician at Makerere University Teaching Hospital, Kampala, Uganda. He helped write the sections on coronary heart disease, diabetes and obesity. He also assisted with research and checking.

I would also like to thank Dr Jim Anderson of Lexington, Kentucky for helpful comments he has made during the revision of this book.

I acknowledge with gratitude the help I have so generously received from literally hundreds of doctors, the majority serving in mission hospitals in Africa and Asia. In spite of perpetual overwork they have always been prepared to take on even more by collecting facts for me which, when strung together like beads on a string, contributed greatly to the formation of the ideas presented in this book.

I would also like to thank Surgeon Captain T.L. Cleave, formerly of the British Navy, who first introduced me to the concept that many of our characteristically Western diseases might be largely the result of the food we eat.

My warmest thanks go to Mrs Sheila King for secretarial and other assistance. And finally I am deeply grateful for the unstinting assistance and helpful advice given by my publisher, Martin Dunitz.

The Publishers would like to thank: Arthur Guinness Son & Co Ltd, London, for permission to reproduce the photograph used for the frontispiece; ICI for permission to reproduce the two photographs by Lennart Nilsson of coronary arteries on page 75; Her Majesty's Stationery Office, London, for permission to reproduce the information contained in the table on page 120 and derived from McCance and Widdowson's *The Composition of Foods*, fourth revised edition by A.A. Paul and D.A.T. Southgate published in 1978. The figure for brown, unpolished rice given on page 120 was supplied by Dr Southgate personally and based on one test. The figure for soya flour was derived from other sources.

INDEX